HYPNOTHERAPY
Is it for you?

Roger Sleet

ELEMENT BOOKS

© Roger Sleet 1988

First published 1983
This edition first published in Great Britain 1988 by
Element Books Limited
Longmead, Shaftesbury, Dorset

Printed and bound in Great Britain by
Billings, Hylton Road, Worcester

Designed by Max Fairbrother

Cover illustration by Ariane Dixon

British Library Cataloguing in Publication Data
Sleet, Roger
Hypnotherapy : is it for you?
1. Medicine, Hypnotherapy
I. Title
615.8'512

ISBN 1-85230-046-9

*This book is dedicated to all those people
who, through no fault of their own, are forced
to suffer discomfort in the belief that
they cannot be cured, when in fact
a cure may be possible*

Contents

Acknowledgements

This book would not have been possible had I not learnt the techniques of hypnotherapy in the first place. My thanks are therefore due to The Institute of Curative Hypnotherapists for the basic training I received from them.

I would also like to thank Mr Stockley of The Institute of Curative Hypnotherapists for his approval and endorsement of this book, and for the Introduction he has written for it.

Most of all, I offer my thanks to the many patients I have treated, who are a walking testimony to the value of this amazing technique, and who gave me an awareness of the need for this book to be written.

Foreword

The practice of hypnosis and the suggestibility that one person has upon another is something that is as old as mankind itself, and many books have been written upon the subject from different viewpoints. Now, at last, we have a book written for the lay person, the man in the street who suddenly hears about hypnotherapy, and now wonders what it's all about. In the past, he has been able to go to a library, collect a book, and read about the achievements and boasts of one hypnotherapist on how he has overcome many ailments and illnesses, but never why he overcame it or how these things occurred.

This book, written by Roger Sleet, is indeed a pleasant change from the rest. Any lay person, with no knowledge whatsoever of hypnosis, will be able to pick it up, read it, and answer many of the questions that they have asked themselves. Why things go wrong, how they go wrong and how one can put them right. It is also a very pleasant change to find that the author has gone out of his way to study not just one aspect of the mind's actions, but to actually take up and acquire a university degree and practice in a clinic situation. In this way he has the practical knowledge, the theoretical knowledge and the ability to compare the conventional disciplines of psychotherapy, psychiatry, and psychology with what is termed a fringe medicine, hypnotherapy. It is very refreshing too that this person can put all these learned subjects together and still feel that the oldest one of all is still the most effective when it comes to assisting mankind in its way through life.

As President of the Institute of Curative Hypnotherapists, I have no hesitation in putting our Institute's form of approval on this book and its publication. I feel that this will make another major step forward into the realms of educating people in a very successful but natural therapeutic means to overcome many of their problems. You will find that this book is not trying to claim miracle cures or anything else. It is not trying to say that hypnotherapy is the answer to everything because this would be unrealistic. What it is trying to point out is that many illnesses, apart from those with a purely bacteriological or viral basis, can originate within one's self. Thus it follows that the illness can be self-motivated and self-destroyed.

This book, in its own way, is going to try and show the lay person how this can come about, and how, with the correct kind of guidance and direction, these things can be corrected and the body can begin to function as nature intended. You will find one or two of the stress-related illnesses mentioned. An unnatural situation brings about unnatural results. On reading this book, I was very pleased to see that the author was not boasting about his own successes in the field of hypnotherapy or trying to claim any rights of ownership or specialisation. It is written on the subject as he sees it, as he compares it with other subjects that he has studied and been involved in. He has put it in simple terms that the lay person can fully understand, so that they can, if necessary, obtain guidance through this very special therapy.

June 1983

R. STOCKLEY
President of the Institute of
Curative Hypnotherapists

Introduction

Nowadays, it is becoming more and more common to look at the "Personal Services" column in a newspaper and find inserts which advertise the services of "Hypnotherapists". Because of restrictions placed on such advertisers by Advertising Standards Authorities, such adverts should contain only business-card details. It therefore follows that whoever reads such an advert must understand just what hypnotherapy is, and what it can do, in order to appreciate just what the service is that is being offered. As this is the case, it also follows that there must be a considerable number of people who could derive benefit from hypnotherapy, but do not do so, simply because they are totally unaware of the facts. In many cases, they do not even know that their condition can be treated by this means.

This book has been written in an attempt to do something about this situation. I hope that after reading this book, the reader will have a clear idea of what hypnotherapy is, and how it may be of use to them. Also included are some useful guides on how to choose a good therapist.

Every attempt has been made to make this book readable to the general public. Medical jargon, wherever possible, has been avoided. Some of the more appropriate or interesting cases have been quoted. In other words, *this book has been written for the patients rather than for the practitioners.*

In the chapters that follow, you will learn a little about the thought behind hypnotherapy, about hypnosis, therapeutic techniques, and their uses. I hope too, you will learn caution, but not a caution based upon a fear of the technique or its effects. More appropriate would be a caution based upon an awareness of the fact that you could, inadvertently, place yourself in the hands of a charlatan. Some hints on how to avoid this situation have also been included.

The above, in a nutshell, is a declaration of the author's intent. Along with this goes my sincere wish that you, the reader, will both learn from and enjoy this book.

How does your brain work?

This question has bothered mankind since he came into being. As yet, no-one has come up with the answer. We have learnt a lot about various aspects of the brain's activity, but even so, we have hardly scratched the surface.

Attempts are continuously being made by psychologists and psychiatrists to offer explanations for our behaviour in terms of what seems to go on in the brain, but the brain is such a complicated organ that such explanations rarely go without opposition. There are times when we seem to have the answer to one of the many questions involved in this problem, but then research suddenly discovers something new which immediately destroys that answer. So a new answer is then offered which will accommodate the new findings.

This seems to be the way of research. An idea is only acceptable until it is disproved. That idea is then modified to include the new findings. It thus becomes nearer to the truth. As this process continues, each successive idea becomes an improvement on its predecessor. Taken to its logical conclusion, the final idea in the chain should be the truth.

In doing their work, researchers often try to produce what they call a "model". A model is a way of explaining what their research leads them to believe is happening in the brain under certain conditions. Models can take many forms. They can be complicated computer programs which attempt to reconstruct the brain's activity, or they can be a simple block diagram, or they can take a variety of other forms.

Every researcher hopes that his model is the right one, but at this stage in the game such an occurrence is unlikely. Models, therefore, are simply expressions of ideas. They should be viewed in this way. Each model indicates at least an element of truth, and does offer some form of explanation which can be used in the development of new research methods, new techniques and new treatments. The knowledge gained from these new models leads to improvements in these fields.

Bearing this in mind, a model will now be presented to you. This model is not offered as established fact, but as an explanation which will help you to understand, in general terms, how your brain may work. If you think of this model when reading about hypnotherapy in later chapters, it will deepen your understanding of the topic.

Let us begin at the beginning. Man is an organism that lives in an environment. From that environment, he receives stimuli, to which he responds. In this case, man responds either physically, mentally, or both physically and mentally. We can show this in the form of a diagram (see Fig. 1).

At this point we can say "so far so good" because this fits the facts as we all see them. So now let us complicate the issue a little. Let us assume that the mediator between the stimulus and the response is the brain and the nervous system. In other words, our mental and physical reactions are simply the product of the brain's behaviour. We need, therefore, to assume something about the brain, and here we enter the realms of theory.

Let us begin by considering the things we do consciously. We use conscious effort, for instance, to think, to reason, to question, to argue and to initiate action. Whenever we use conscious effort, we are aware of it. So let us sum up these activities and say that they are all governed by the activity of the "conscious mind"

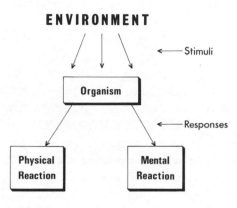

Fig. 1

Now let us consider some of the things we do subconsciously. This is necessary because some of the things we do require no conscious effort at all – we do them automatically. Consider walking, for instance. Do you know which foot you start with? Do you know how many paces you take? You don't, because all you do is consciously initiate the action, and then everything else that happens is automatic. The same is true of talking. When you talk, you don't think about vocabulary, grammar, sentence construction, or any of these things. You just talk. How do we explain this?

The easiest way is to consider what we have done. Throughout our lives, we have learnt to do certain things so well that we no longer have to think about them. When we first began to learn these things, it took a lot of conscious effort. When we first learnt to walk, we were only too aware of what each foot was doing. The activity required our fullest attention, and was therefore under the control of the conscious mind. But as we became more skilled, the conscious mind became less involved, until eventually it was not involved at all, except to initiate the action. It was as though it was slowly being transferred from the conscious mind to some other part of the brain. So let us call this other part the "subconscious mind", and we will include in there anything that we don't do consciously.

This, of course, means that the subconscious mind is far more complex than the conscious mind, because, as we have already indicated, the brain also governs us physically, as well as mentally. Consider, for instance, what happens when we go to sleep at night. The moment we drift into sleep, we lose all consciousness. It is as though our conscious minds have ceased to exist. Yet throughout the night our hearts keep beating, our lungs expand and contract, chemical reactions continue within our body. In short, we are kept alive by the normal operation of our body functions. But what controls them? Again, it is the brain. So we'll include this kind of function as part of the job of the subconscious mind.

We have now succeeded in dividing the brain into two convenient parts: the conscious and the subconscious. Now to use our common sense to try to build up a more detailed model. We can do this by elaborating on our first model. As we do this, the questions we ask will help to fill the model out.

In order to respond to a stimulus, it must first be perceived. Our first question therefore, is "what perceives it?" Is it the conscious or the subconscious?

As we go through our daily lives, we continuously search our surroundings for information. Frequently, we use the ability to focus all our attention on just one sense, as, for instance, when listening to music. We may close our eyes in order to concentrate more on the music. This is a conscious action. We do it in order to gain a better perception of the stimulus. We can therefore say that stimuli from the environment are perceived by the conscious mind.

However, not all stimuli are perceived consciously. Imagine for a moment that you are asleep in your bed. At some time during the night the temperature of the room changes, so that the room becomes much colder. What happens? There comes a point where you wake up *because you feel cold*. But in order for this to happen, that coldness must have been perceived subconsciously because we were not aware of it until we woke up. We must therefore conclude that stimuli are also perceived by the subconscious mind.

Having established that both the conscious and the subconscious are capable of perceiving stimuli from the environment, let us now consider the question of responses to those stimuli. Our original model indicated that we can respond physically, mentally, or both physically and mentally. We now need to know what contribution the two minds make to these responses.

In this respect, the conscious mind is quickly dealt with. If you are asked a question, you think about it, reason it out, and give a reply. The thinking and reasoning is done with full awareness, and is therefore a conscious mental response. Giving a verbal reply requires the manipulation of the mouth and vocal cords, etc., and this is therefore a conscious physical response. So we quickly conclude that the conscious mind can respond both physically and mentally.

In discussing the responses of the subconscious mind, it is useful to consider one of the stimuli that we can receive from the environment, and that is stress. Stress takes many forms, but in this instance let us imagine that you suddenly find yourself in a very dangerous position. Under these conditions, a very special part of the nervous system comes into action without any conscious control. As a result of this, you produce adrenalin, which causes your pupils to dilate, your mouth to go dry, your heartbeat to speed up, and the blood supply to your muscles to increase. This reaction prepares your body for action so that you are more able to cope with the situation. If these physical changes are not brought about consciously, then it follows that the subconscious mind must be able to produce a physical response.

Stress can also affect our mental state. Conditions like depression, anxiety and apathy are all reactions to stress. These conditions are not produced consciously in most cases. Although it is possible to do so, one normally does not consciously attempt to produce depression, for instance. It must therefore be a subconscious response of a mental nature.

We have now reached a point where we can say that stimuli received from the environment can be perceived both by the conscious and the subconscious minds. Added to this, we can now say that the conscious and the subconscious minds can respond to these stimuli both physically and mentally. But the picture is not yet complete. We must now ask whether the two minds work in isolation or whether they are connected. In order to answer this question, let us consider the aspect of memory.

When we try to remember things, there are degrees of success or failure in how well we can do it. Some things we can remember clearly and well, while other things we cannot remember at all. Sometimes we can work at trying to remember something, and after a period of time it suddenly comes to us. How can we explain this?

Let us assume that as events happen to us, they are recorded in some sort of memory bank. There they are stored until required for further use. Remembering is simply withdrawing an item from that memory bank.

Our first question is "Where is that memory bank located?" If it were located in the conscious mind, we would not have to work in order to find certain memories, and even if we did, we would always succeed. It must therefore be located in the subconscious mind.

However, because of the way we use our memories, we have to conclude that the conscious mind must have access to the memory bank. There is therefore a connecting link from the conscious mind to the subconscious mind.

Similarly, we know that there must also be a link from the subconscious to the conscious. There are occasions, for instance, when for no apparent reason a memory will suddenly be called into consciousness. This can happen under many circumstances, even when engrossed in conversation with someone else. The subconscious mind has fed that memory to the conscious mind. This it could not do if that link did not exist.

Now we are ready to produce our model, and this we have done in Fig. 2. You will see that all the links we have discussed are shown on this model, and it will help to clarify some of the points made in later chapters.

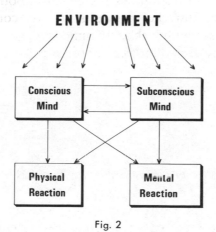

Fig. 2

It should be stated here that this model would probably infuriate many academics, who would declare it as too simplistic, or even positively wrong. But this would be missing the point. This model is not put forward as proven scientific fact, but as a means of helping you, as the reader, to understand what is going on in your brain. If you have a problem, you may already be thinking of it in terms of this model, thinking how your problem fits into this picture. If so, you are taking the right approach.

2

What is hypnosis?

Hypnosis, obviously, is the medium through which the hypnotherapist works. But in order to appreciate what a hypnotherapist does, one also needs to understand what hypnosis is, and why it is of value in terms of our model.

In order to appreciate this, we first need to know something about consciousness and unconsciousness.

If you think for a moment about your own experience of consciousness, you will easily appreciate that it is not always the same. Sometimes you will be wide awake, alert, and on form. At other times you will be more sluggish and less alert. Sometimes you will be positively daydreamy. These conditions are all different and can be represented as different "levels" of consciousness. If you imagine yourself standing on a staircase, when you are standing on the top stair, then let that represent yourself at your most awake. As you descend the stairs, each successive stair represents a state where you are less alert, slower, and more daydreamy.

Naturally, as you continue to descend, you will soon reach a point where you are hardly awake at all, and a further step will take you into sleep itself. A loss of consciousness. An entry into unconsciousness.

Sleep, like consciousness, has levels. There is deep sleep, light sleep, and other levels in between. It is as though that staircase continues to go down and down into the deepest possible state of sleep.

We therefore have a continuum which ranges from full consciousness to complete unconsciousness, like a long staircase. Throughout the twenty-four hours of your day, your position on that staircase changes according to your current state of consciousness.

Now this all seems very straightforward and simple. It seems to cover everything, and in a way it does.

If we now think about hypnosis, it does not complicate this continuum, it fits into it. This is shown in Fig. 3. As you will see from this diagram, hypnosis also has levels. At some levels the subject is conscious and aware, while at other levels the subject is unconscious. It is therefore during hypnosis that the transformation from being awake to being asleep takes place.

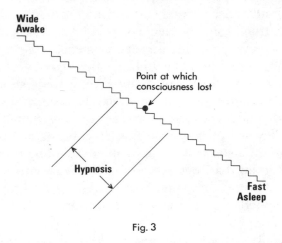

Fig. 3

Looked at in this way, you can easily see that there is nothing magical or mysterious about hypnosis. In fact it is a natural condition that you pass through at least twice each day: you pass through it in order to awaken from sleep, and you pass through it again in order to go to sleep. In the normal way of things the passage through hypnosis is quick and uneventful. Because of this we hardly notice its passing. So why is this part of the continuum so important?

Let us refer back to our model at this point. If we think about the conscious mind, then we can easily see that we only have access to it on the upper half of the continuum, i.e. when we are awake. But what about the subconscious mind? It helps here to think of the subconscious mind as being like a safe. The contents of that safe are protected behind the safe door. During our waking hours, that door remains tightly shut, unless we wish to put something into it or take something out of it. In this way our habits remain secure and unaffected by outside influences.

However, during sleep, this security is relaxed a little, as though the safe door were partly open. This was demonstrated with the old technique of "sleep learning". If you wished to learn something well, then it was recorded on tape. A tape recorder with a timing device was placed at the bedside, with the speaker in the pillow. You would simply set the timer and go to sleep. At the specified time the tape recorder would switch on and play the tape to you while asleep. On awakening, you would find that you had a much better grasp of the subject being learnt. For this to have occurred, there must have been some access to the subconscious mind.

From this we can see that in consciousness we have little or no access to the subconscious mind, but in sleep we have more access to it. Hypnosis, however, is a little different.

During hypnosis, it is as though that safe door swings wide open. There is a direct access to the subconscious mind in its entirety. This allows information to be put in and taken out with little or no difficulty.

This simple fact carries enormous implications, particularly when we consider just what that subconscious mind contains. Suppose, for instance, that you wish to break a habit, like smoking. It simply means that you implant

some information in the subconscious mind which will
enable you to achieve this easily, with no craving, no loss of
temper, no substitution (like eating sweets, etc.), and a
feeling of well-being.

Of course, this is a simple example, so let us now consider
something more complicated. Suppose this time that you
suffer from a fear, a phobia. Most phobias have an origin,
usually an event which may have taken place many years
ago and is now forgotten. The access to the subconscious
also means access to the memory bank. So we can search
that memory bank to find the cause of the phobia. From this
we can find out what the brain did in order to produce the
phobic reaction. Thus we can find out the history of the
condition. Having done this, we can then replace the exist-
ing procedure with a new procedure which does away with
fear.

These two examples serve to demonstrate the value of
hypnosis, and by now you may already be thinking to yourself in terms of these concepts. More will be said about this
later, but first, let us concentrate on hypnosis.

I have talked about hypnosis as being part of the "consciousness continuum". All that happens during the hypnotic process is that you are led to that part of the
continuum and held there for a while. It is while you are
held in this continuum that the work is done. I will now try
to describe this condition.

As I have already stated, there are levels of hypnosis, and
just as your experience of consciousness changes as you
progress from wakefulness to drowsiness, so too the experience of hypnosis changes from the lighter states to the
deeper states.

In a light trance state, you would probably find that your
eyes were closed, but that you were more aware of your
surroundings than usual. You would notice any faint noises
that may occur, and distant noises would seem much nearer.
Because of this awareness you might think that you could

just get up and do something else, and indeed you could.

The only reason you don't do it is because you are happy to stay where you are. You feel comfortable and relaxed. But it's too much trouble to get up anyway. So you stay where you are. Light states like this are very deceiving because although your eyes are closed, everything else seems perfectly normal, and in this condition you can actually fool yourself into believing that you are not hypnotised when in fact you are.

As the trance state deepens, you become less aware of your surroundings. You could reach a stage where awareness seems to come and go. At this point you are on the threshold of losing consciousness, thus beginning to enter the lower half of the consciousness continuum.

Beyond this point you enter the states which we call "somnambulism". These states can only be described as being like sleep itself. All awareness is gone.

At this point it is good to remember that we are talking about people, and people are individuals. If you were to go to a hypnotherapist for treatment, he would induce hypnosis artificially. He would use his techniques to induce this state in you. Quite naturally, you would probably feel a little apprehensive at your first encounter with hypnosis. This apprehension would not prevent you from responding, but it might well affect the depth of trance you achieve. It is therefore very possible that you would only achieve a light state. But this does not mean that you cannot achieve a greater depth. You can learn this through practice, just as practice improves performance when learning, for instance, to play the piano.

As you read the above, you may be comparing this with what you have seen on the stage or television. If so, you will already have decided that the people you saw were in a state of somnambulism, and you would be right. Does this therefore mean that a stage hypnotist is more adept at hypnosis than a hypnotherapist? No, and for a very good reason. So let us now discuss the differences between stage hypnosis and hypnotherapy.

A stage hypnotist makes use of one very important fact, and that is that about 10% of the population as a whole are very special people as far as hypnosis is concerned. With such people, their response to hypnosis is unique. They immediately become somnambulistic. They lose all awareness, and on awakening they have no idea of what happened while in the trance. These people are indeed special, but there are not many of them about.

The stage hypnotist is very aware of this, and he has been trained to locate these people in an audience. Without such people he would not be able to put on such an impressive exhibition. He therefore knows that in an audience of, say, two thousand, there may be 200 people he can use. There is no way he could simply take the front row and use them because he knows that they would not respond to his approach, unless of course they were somnambulists. Using this piece of information, a stage hypnotist can put on a good show and leave a deep impression on his audience.

The hypnotherapist, on the other hand, gains no benefit from this information. He is faced with the prospect of having to be able to hypnotise every patient that enters the door. He is therefore concerned with the other 90% of the population as well as the somnambulists. His techniques are therefore different. He appreciates that he is dealing with people who cannot enter a somnambulistic state with a click of the fingers, or something similar.

In other words, the two situations are entirely different. Even a somnambulist who visits a hypnotherapist is likely to lose that somnambulistic response on that occasion. His problem will prevent it happening.

It is very important that this difference be realised. So many people base their expectations upon their impressions of stage hypnosis, and this is a fatal mistake to make. What you see on stage is something special. It does not represent hypnosis as a whole.

Another false impression that arises from stage hypnosis is that of the Svengali image. By this one means the idea that the hypnotist is the master, and the subject his slave. Nothing could be further from the truth. At all times it is the subject that decides what he will or will not do. He will only carry out an order that he is not in opposition to. Any instruction that goes against the subject's principles will not be carried out. In fact, it will not be carried out even if he simply does not want to do it.

Why then, one might ask, do the people on stage carry out acts like crowing like a rooster? There are two reasons. Firstly, it does not offend their principles to do so. Such an act is not something one feels strongly about. Secondly, and more importantly, the explanation given to the subject for doing so seems to make sense. More will be said about this later, but for now it is enough to say that the decision to act or not to act can be influenced if sufficient reason is given by the hypnotist.

Hypnosis then, does not take away your willpower. Nor does it take away your freedom to think or make decisions. You remain a completely free agent, and you decide what you will or will not do. In fact, rather than take anything away from you, hypnosis tends to give to you heightened abilities.

In that trance state, several things happen. The most widely known thing is that you become very suggestible. Things tend to make more sense while in hypnosis than they would in full consciousness. Part of this is due to the fact that your imagination also comes alive. Under hypnosis, you can imagine something to the extent that it seems to be a reality. For instance, if you were asked to imagine that your leg was embedded in concrete, then to you, that concrete would be so real that you would be unable to move your foot. This suggestibility and the use of the imagination is true at all levels of hypnosis.

At deeper levels, you are able to do more things. You can, for instance, remember things that have long since been forgotten. It is, in fact, possible to remember in detail your birth. (More will be said about this in the chapter on regression.) This being the case, it is easy to see how it becomes possible to establish how a phobia, for example, began.

From this it can be seen that with problems which can be dealt with simply by using direct suggestions, a light trance will do. In order to find out certain things, a deeper trance is necessary. It therefore follows that the level of hypnosis determines which techniques can or cannot be used. If you have a problem which requires that the therapist must get you to remember far back into the past, then it is highly unlikely that this will be attempted on your first visit. You will need practice in order to achieve the required depth of trance.

At this point it may be advisable to say that many people get worried at the prospect of remembering past events. If this is true of you, the following may be of some comfort. It has been the experience of the author that many conditions result from the first five years of life. This may, of course, just be a coincidence. However, if such were to be the case, one must remember that one used the reasoning of an infant to fathom out that event. To the mind of a child, that event may have been devastating, while to an adult it would be insignificant. It is often, therefore surprising to the patient to learn that such an event should cause such problems in later life, simply because they can now use adult reasoning to understand the event. The ordeal of regression in such cases is no ordeal at all.

However, there are cases where the event is horrific. The therapist will obviously appreciate this. In such cases, there are steps which can be taken. For instance, you could be instructed to go completely to sleep and awaken with no recall of what happened during the treatment session. Added to this will be suggestions that on awakening you will feel happy and relaxed and even relieved. In short, no therapist worth his salt will allow you to awaken feeling any ill effects from such a session.

Let us now go on to the subject of "things that can go wrong". Basically, very little can go wrong with this technique, and even if it does it is not disastrous. Most therapists issue cassette tapes to their patients which include a hypnotic induction. In other words, listening to that tape will hypnotise you. These tapes are used in order to reinforce the treatment. So let us assume for a moment that you are playing that tape and you are hypnotised, when suddenly, through no fault of your own, something happens. Perhaps there is a power cut, or the tape breaks. The obvious question is "What happens to you?"

In such a case there are only two possibilities. The most likely is that you will immediately wake up, wondering why it has gone quiet, but suffering no other ill effects. The only other possibility is that you could drift into a natural sleep and awaken later, in your own time. There is no way that you will spend the rest of your life in a trance! Which of these two occurs is often determined by your state of mind at the time. If you feel tired, you will probably go to sleep. If not, you will probably awaken. In other words, nothing harmful can result from such a disaster, other than perhaps a feeling of disappointment. In any case, such events are rare in the extreme.

On very rare occasions, a patient will awaken and complain of a headache, or dizziness. If this should happen to you, then you should tell the therapist immediately. He will then quickly put you back into the trance and give you suggestions that will take it away and prevent it happening again. But once again, this is extremely rare.

Hopefully, by now you have a much clearer idea of what hypnosis is, and of what to expect if you find yourself on the receiving end of a hypnotic induction. Be assured that it is safe, and that nothing harmful can happen to you. It is a natural state, and a valuable state. It can be used to help you with a considerable number of problems, as I will now discuss.

3

Special cases of hypnosis

In the previous chapter, I have discussed hypnosis in terms of levels. The levels discussed are those which one would expect to experience in the hypnotherapist's consulting room. However, there are other levels which can be broadly categorised under the heading of "waking hypnosis".

Waking hypnosis is found at the "conscious end" of the hypnosis continuum. At this level, the subject's eyes are open and is almost fully conscious. It is therefore difficult to describe. So let us consider an example.

Some years ago, there was a patient who had great difficulty whenever he had to visit a dentist. Whenever the dentist tried to put anything in his mouth the patient would retch violently. Dental appointments would usually end with a red–faced patient with tears running down his face, and a frustrated and exasperated dentist. Eventually, it reached a point where the only way the patient could have treatment was by using a general anaesthetic.

Later on, the patient moved to a new county, and therefore lost touch with his dentist. The time came when he needed dental treatment again, and he went in search of a dentist who used general anaesthesia. The first dentist he tried listened sympathetically as he described his problem. The dentist then suggested that he could use a technique which would not involve anaesthesia at all, and there was no reason why this should not work for this patient.

The patient was asked to clasp his hands together with his

fingers interlocked, and to grip hard. He was to concentrate all his attention on his hands and keep that grip firm. After a few seconds of this, the patient was asked to settle down and open his mouth, but to keep concentrating on that grip. The dentist began to work. The patient did not retch. After a few minutes, the patient was allowed to relax his grip and make his hands comfortable while the dentist continued his work. The end result of this was that the dentist was able to complete his treatment successfully, and the patient did not retch once during the entire treatment.

That patient learnt from this experience, and on each occasion when he required dental treatment he would carry out this ritual by himself, with the result that he was never bothered by that problem again.

What happened here was that the patient's attention was diverted away from the fact that the dentist was working in his mouth. He was thinking about something else, and concentrating hard upon it. While he was doing this, the dentist simply suggested that there would be no discomfort while he worked. The patient accepted this suggestion and responded to it. The situation became real simply because the suggestion made it so.

This was an example of waking hypnosis, and as you can see, although it is a simple approach, it is also a very powerful one.

Perhaps at this point you may like to try a small experiment yourself. Just read the next paragraph slowly and carefully, and think about it as you read.

Try this for yourself now. Just think about the act of swallowing. Concentrate upon that thought. If you do this, you will find it impossible not to go through with it, even though you may try to resist it. In fact, if you try to resist it, you will feel a great sense of unease. You want to swallow. You can feel it now. Your mouth is filling with saliva as you read this. You really want to swallow don't you? In fact, you are just going to have to swallow, aren't you? Well, aren't you?

Now this may or may not have worked with you, but if it did, you accepted the suggestions and put them into effect even though you were only reading. If you did not respond to this, now ask yourself whether or not you have swallowed since reading the paragraph. The chances are that you have. Response does not have to be immediate. It can have a kind of delayed reaction. Of course, you can argue that swallowing is a natural function that occurs at frequent intervals anyway. But if you feel that this is what happened, do it again, but try to control it this time.

If you found that you were unable to respond to this, then do not take it as an indication that you cannot be hypnotised. This example is simply included because most people can respond to it, but not necessarily everyone. More is said about this in later chapters.

It is, however, a good example of waking hypnosis. If you did swallow, then you accepted the suggestion even though you were fully conscious. This is what makes waking hypnosis a special case – it can occur during full consciousness.

This, of course, leads to some interesting questions about advertising. We are all subjected to advertising techniques in a variety of ways. This can be through television, magazines, newspapers, hoardings, etc. We can therefore ask whether a subtle form of waking hypnosis is involved here. The simple answer is "yes". To some extent, the repetitive nature of advertising ensures that the name of the product is continuously suggested to us. This means that if we wish to buy, for instance, a tin of baked beans, then one particular make will immediately come into our minds.

Let us now turn to another special case of hypnosis. In our discussion so far, we have been concerned with hypnosis as a condition which can be induced in us by an outside influence, such as a hypnotherapist. It is, however, possible for you to induce this condition in yourself without any outside help. This is a technique which can be learnt easily and quickly, and it is becoming increasingly popular in its use, particularly by such as students who wish to improve their study activities and examination performance.

Self-hypnosis enables the subject to give himself suggestions which will enable him to achieve a particular goal. In order to do this, the subject induces a trance state in himself, in order to open up a channel of communication to the subconscious mind.

Obviously, the trance state must be one of the lighter states, in order that the subject is conscious enough to be able to give himself suggestions. He would be unable to do this if he were to enter a somnambulistic state.

Self-hypnosis is also demonstrated by the case of the dental patient discussed earlier. Later on, that patient changed his dentist again. The new dentist did not understand or appreciate the technique that had been used. He insisted that the patient just act like a normal patient, with the result that the patient retched. Eventually, the dentist was asked to allow the patient to carry out the procedure he had learnt. This he did successfully, with the result that the dentist was able to complete his task successfully.

In this instance, the patient had handled the whole affair by himself. He simply gave himself the necessary suggestions and was able to bring about the desired result.

Here, of course, the patient induced a state of waking hypnosis in himself. It is, however, possible to induce in yourself a deeper level of hypnosis using different procedures.

Waking hypnosis and self-hypnosis are discussed here as special cases of hypnosis. But they are only special in so far as they are generally used for special purposes. Whereas a dentist, for instance, will use waking hypnosis to a large extent, a hypnotherapist only uses it as a side issue. Similarly, self-hypnosis can be taught by a hypnotherapist, but is not an integral part of the treatment. Since this book is primarily concerned with hypnotherapy, these two cases are therefore set apart as special, and are not discussed in greater detail.

At this point, it is appropriate to make a seemingly contradictory statement. When it really comes down to it, all hypnosis is self-induced. This is because it is you that follows the suggestions that lead you into the trance state. The hypnotist has no unseen power. There is no magic or mysticism involved. In fact, if you wished not to be hypnotised, then you could easily resist the suggestions. In this case, you would remain fully conscious. It therefore follows, that by freely accepting the suggestions and acting upon them, it is you that puts yourself into the trance state.

The term "self-hypnosis" is therefore used here only to apply to the situation where you intentionally, and with full awareness, induce that state in yourself.

4

Can you be hypnotised?

There are many people who will not go to see a hypno-therapist simply because they believe that they cannot be hypnotised. Let us therefore look a little closer at this question of who can, and who cannot be hypnotised.

As you read the previous chapters, you may already have found that the descriptions may not fit the conceptions you had of hypnosis. However, it is a common failing of man that his preconceived ideas become hard and fast, and they are not easily dislodged. This is exemplified by the fact that no matter how hard one tries to explain to a new patient that he will not "go to sleep", most patients still expect this to happen. It is not until they actually experience it and see its effects that they finally accept the explanation.

The belief that one cannot be hypnotised is no exception to this principle. The idea can be used as a protection. It is sometimes a comforting thought to believe that it cannot happen to you. But what happens if you are suffering with a problem that you know hypnotherapy can cure? That comforting belief can then be a problem to you. It can even reach the point where you think that since you cannot be hypnotised, then it is pointless to go for treatment. You therefore decide that you will just have to put up with the problem and learn to live with it. But is this decision correct? What really is the truth of the matter?

Let us look a little more closely at the facts.

Throughout the years, there has been a considerable

amount of research done on this very question. The findings of a number of projects have been expressed in terms of the percentage of the population which cannot be hypnotised. However, if you collect all these findings together and compare them, you find a considerable amount of disagreement between them, i.e. the percentage of the population which cannot be hypnotised ranges from about 3% to about 66%.

Obviously, with discrepancies of this size, such findings must be treated with suspicion. Rather than say that those people *cannot* be hypnotised, it would be better to say that they were not hypnotised *on that occasion*. This enables us to ask why.

From our earlier discussion, we already know that it is possible to resist a hypnotic induction. In fact, it is very easy to do this. It is even easier if you are not happy with the therapist or the conditions under which he works. From this you can see that there are other factors involved in hypnosis besides the patient himself. Just imagine yourself being shown into a cold and clinical consulting room, that seems to be designed to make you feel uncomfortable, and then being confronted by an officious bully of a therapist. Are you likely to give your fullest co-operation under these circumstances? Of course not. The strength of your own feelings will make you hold back.

It is not being suggested that this is what happened during this research, but it is highly possible that some elements of this were present on these occasions, and this could have influenced the results. It is also possible that the hypnotists were inexperienced, and that their techniques were not appropriate for the patients. In fact, there are an enormous number of factors which could have led to this variation in these results.

Obviously then, we cannot look to research for an answer to the question. Let us therefore be a little more down-to-earth in our approach.

If we look at the problem logically, we soon reach the conclusion that if a hypnotherapist could not hypnotise 66% of his patients, then 66% of his time would be wasted, and he could not survive. If this were the case, it would also mean that there would be a decrease in interest in hypnotherapy, rather than the increase in interest that exists at the moment, and the increase in acceptance by the medical profession. We can therefore immediately dismiss a percentage of such large proportions.

On the other hand, a proportion of 3% would be much more acceptable. At this point you could say: "Ah yes. But I am one of the 3%". But would you be right?

Let us ask a few pertinent questions here. What makes you say that? Are you any different from any other human? You are built in the same way. You have a brain, like anyone else. It has the same bits and pieces that all brains have. If others can be hypnotised, but you can't, then they have something that is missing in you. Are you therefore saying that there is some part of your brain that doesn't work as it should? If hypnosis is as natural as we say, then why can't you perform a natural function?

Suddenly, the inability to be hypnotised is not so comforting a thought, is it?

Perhaps it is a question of skill then. Perhaps the mechanisms are there, but you have simply never learnt to use them. But then, neither has any patient that comes for treatment for the first time, and yet they can do it very successfully with no prior experience. So why can't you?

If you believe you cannot be hypnotised, then dwell on these thoughts for a moment. When it really comes down to it, isn't it simply that you have clung on to this idea simply to protect yourself because the thought of being hypnotised is worrying to you? Is it not more a question of the fact that you feel you would be "handing over control" to somebody else, and that this is something you do not feel you can bring yourself to do?

Look at this a little more closely. Just think of other times in your life when you had to "hand over control". You must have visited a dentist at some time in your life, or a doctor. You may even have had an operation. Did you have any control over these situations? Even if you ride on a bus or a train or fly in an aeroplane, you are placing your life in the hands of the driver, or pilot. Again, you have no control. If any of these people had, for instance, a heart attack while performing their tasks, what could you do? Nothing, because you have placed yourself in their hands. *They* have control. What you are in fact doing here is using their skills to help you to achieve some goal. In these cases, to improve your health or to reach a destination. You hand over control in order that you may benefit from their skills.

By the same token, if you know that a hypnotherapist has skills which can be of benefit to you in overcoming a problem, would it not be foolish not to hand over control, particularly since you have already done it several times in your life?

More important still is the fact that the question of "control" does not even enter into the argument, because at all times *you* are in control. Think about the dental patient we discussed in the previous chapter. Who was controlling him? He was, of course, controlling himself. The dentist simply showed him how to do it. Hypnosis does *not* take away your willpower, or anything else. You still have the freedom to think, and to make decisions. You are a completely free agent at all times. If a suggestion were given to you that went against your principles, you simply would not accept it. Even if you simply did not want to accept it, you would still reject it. So even though hypnotised, you still have full control.

It is in this principle that the anwer to our question lies. It is not a question of whether or not you can be hypnotised. Rather, it is a question of whether or not you will allow yourself to be hypnotised.

In reality, the only people who *cannot* be hypnotised are those who suffer from a mental condition which will not allow them to concentrate for more than one or two sentences at a time. Such people are usually institutionalised. Other people who do not enter the trance state are holding themselves back.

On occasions, the idea that one cannot be hypnotised comes as a result of some previous encounter with a hypnotherapist when it did not seem to work. So let us now consider this.

A good hypnotherapist will always take the time to explain to you what you should expect. If he does not do this, you may expect the wrong things. You may expect to go to sleep, for instance. If you do not go to sleep, your expectations are not fulfilled. Therefore, you cannot accept that you were hypnotised (even though you may have been), and because of this you reject his suggestions and the treatment fails.

This is one reason which may explain this, but it is not the only reason. As we have already said, there are many factors involved in hypnosis. Sometimes the patient does not like the personality of the therapist, and therefore finds co-operation difficult. Sometimes the patient finds the consulting room uncomfortable. This too is distracting. Sometimes a sound can occur which has particular relevance to the patient and this destroys the induction. All of these things can have brought about the failure on that occasion.

On the question of sounds, usually background noises do not matter. However, to a switchboard operator, for instance, the sound of a telephone ringing is a signal for action, and this could bring about a "reflex action" and bring such a person back to full consciousness. To anyone else, such a sound would be irrelevant and would be ignored. Different people attach different importance to different sounds. Silence has the same effect, and can, in fact, be more distracting. However, distraction caused by sounds or silence is very rare.

If, then, you have tried and failed, do not take this as an indication that you cannot be hypnotised. That would be a wrong conclusion. You may have been unlucky in your choice of therapist. So do not use this as an excuse for not going for treatment. You *can* be hypnotised. Make no mistake about that. The final chapter in this book gives guidance on how to choose a good therapist. So read it, and try again.

How is hypnosis induced?

The task of any hypnotist is to guide the subject to a level of consciousness that is within the range of "hypnotic states". For this to be successful, certain preconditions need to be met.

The role the hypnotist plays is that of guide. He shows his subject the way. The subject, on the other hand, has a choice. He can choose whether or not he wishes to follow those directions. If he resists them, then obviously, he will not be hypnotised. However, if he does choose to follow them, then he will easily achieve that altered state of consciousness. From this it can be seen that the co-operation of the subject is a necessary precondition.

Somnambulists are different. They feel naturally compelled to co-operate, and are therefore the easiest of subjects. However, in the therapeutic situation, even a somnambulist can lose this ability, because their problem can generate a more powerful force which counteracts that natural tendency. One cannot therefore make assumptions on the basis of previous hypnotic experience. Co-operation is needed, even in the case of somnambulists.

It is also necessary that the patient be in agreement with the purpose for which hypnosis is being used. If this is not the case, then all suggestions leading to the achievement of that purpose will be automatically rejected.

If these preconditions are met, then the stage is set for a successful induction.

The main aim of the induction is to bring about a state of complete relaxation in the subject, both physically and mentally. The ways in which this can be done are many and varied. In fact, there are more methods than there are hypnotists.

Some people think of hypnotic procedures as involving such things as swinging pendulums, crystal balls, flashing lights, and so on. Others think in terms of: "look into my eyes". Indeed, it is possible to induce a hypnotic trance using such devices. However, this kind of approach is hardly used at all now. In olden days, a hypnotist would use such things, but this was more important to the production of an air of mystique than it was to the induction of a trance state. Nowadays, the mystique has been swept aside, and more natural methods are used.

Usually, the first thing that happens is that you are made comfortable somewhere. Some therapists will lay you down on a couch or a bed, while others will seat you in a reclining chair or a comfortable armchair. There are also one or two therapists who use vibrating chairs. These give a very pleasant sensation, but they are just a trimming, and are not really necessary.

You will also be asked not to cross your legs or your arms. The reason for this is that the physical relaxation of the limbs is accompanied by a heaviness in those limbs. If they are crossed, they can become very uncomfortable, and since everything is too much trouble in the trance state, it is also too much trouble to uncross them. At the time, the discomfort is no problem, but on awakening from the trance the effects of that discomfort are very strong.

Having got the preliminaries out of the way, the therapist will then proceed with the induction process. This involves giving you a series of suggestions, each of which are designed to play some part in guiding you into a very relaxed trance state.

On average, it takes about ten to fifteen minutes for a new

patient to reach a satisfactory level of hypnosis. During this time, the induction goes through two, or more, stages. The initial induction guides the patient into a very light level of hypnosis. This is followed by one or two deepening processes. Usually, at this point, therapy can begin.

It should be emphasised here that the use of the term "deepening processes" does not mean that you are guided into somnambulism. This will hardly ever happen on the initial encounter with hypnosis. It simply means that the depth of trance is slightly increased to be sure that your level of consciousness is well within the range of hypnotic states.

The initial induction can take many forms, and the therapist will have several approaches available to him. He will have chosen those approaches in order to be able to match his induction to the patient. (e.g. It would be pointless to include suggestions concerning deep breathing if the patient is on a respirator.) A little of the personality of the therapist is involved here, because he will use the approaches that *he* feels comfortable with. If he feels comfortable with it and has confidence in it, then he will have a very fluent delivery which will result in a smooth and successful induction. If he felt uneasy about his technique, his delivery would be full of hesitations, and his uncertainty would be quickly detected by the patient. The patient would therefore lose confidence in the therapist and all would be lost.

It would be impossible, in a book of this size, to discuss the many approaches in great depth. What therefore follows is a very general description of a few of the techniques which can be used.

One of the techniques which can be used involves the therapist naming various parts of the body. As he does this, you tightly flex the muscles in that part of your body, and then release them. With this procedure, you gradually work through your entire body, step by step. The idea of this is to bring about a physical relaxation.

While this can be effective, it also has its setbacks. Patients with certain conditions can find that the flexion of certain muscles will bring about pain, and this will do nothing to promote a state of relaxation. This is also true for some people who wear false teeth. If they are asked to clench their teeth very tightly, it can again be a painful experience. One also has to bear in mind that a patient who, for instance, comes for treatment to stop smoking may also suffer from arthritis. So although such an approach may be fine for the problem being treated, it may not be fine for the other condition which also exists. However, where these conditions do not apply, the approach can be very successful.

Either before or after this procedure, you are asked to close your eyes. When the procedure has been completed, you are then usually asked to imagine something of a relaxing nature. The theory behind this is that now you are physically relaxed, you can now become mentally relaxed too.

Usually, hypnotherapists have good imaginations themselves. They can dream up some beautiful pictures for you to imagine in order to bring about that mental relaxation. It may be a walk in the country or a stroll along the coast. Or it could be something even more simple, like just basking in the sunshine. Whatever the picture, the therapist's powers of description are very much in play. Your attention is drawn to various aspects of the scene, and the feelings you experience as a result of the use of your own imagination.

It is really this part of this approach that does most of the work. The better your imagination, the more successful you are in your response. On completion of this phase, you are now ready for the application of a deepening process. This is covered separately later.

There are, of course, many variations on this theme. Each therapist will add his own twists and turns to this approach, if he uses it at all. He may reverse the procedure, or use some different kind of exercise for the muscles.

Another method which can be used involves the therapist

asking you to concentrate all your attention upon something while he predicts what is going to happen. Included in this is a set of suggestions of a relaxing nature. With this method, there are an amazing number of variations. One or two of these variations are given below.

A particularly impressive variation involves staring at your own hand as it rests, for instance, on the arm of a chair. As you stare at your hand, suggestions are given which direct your attention to various parts of that hand. You are made aware of certain sensations in that hand, including a sensation of lightness. As the process continues, that hand becomes lighter and lighter until it actually lifts itself clear of the arm of the chair. You watch your own hand float up into the air, turn, and begin to approach your face. As soon as any part of that hand touches any part of the face, your eyes immediately close, your hand relaxes and drops to your side again, and you quickly drift into a deeply relaxed condition.

This particular approach is both fascinating to watch and extremely effective. It has much to recommend it. The patient has the evidence of his own eyes to tell him that something is happening. This reinforces his confidence in the ability of the therapist. The result of this is the achievement of a deeper level of hypnosis at the end of the initial induction stage.

With a similar variation, you are asked to hold a weight in your hand, while holding that hand out in front of you. You are asked to position your hand in such a way that you can stick out your thumb horizontally. Thus the back of your hand faces upwards, and the fingers take the weight of the object. You are then asked to stare at your thumbnail, while suggestions are given that the fingers will relax their grip on the object, thus making the hand slowly open. At the point where the object drops out of the hand, again, you close your eyes, your hand drops down, and you drift into a relaxed condition.

While these two variations are different, they share certain things of importance. With both variations, the attention is concentrated upon one specific thing. While the attention is held in this way, the predictive and relaxing suggestions are built up to a climax, at which everything seems to happen all at once.

On a first encounter with this type of approach it is not uncommon to see a look of surprise and disbelief appear on the patient's face as, for instance, the hand begins to rise into the air. However, this quickly disappears as the induction proceeds and they begin to feel more relaxed.

In evaluating this type of method one must acknowledge its effectiveness. However, it does have an important drawback. Extensive use is made these days of cassette tape recordings in therapy. These are of considerable value in reinforcing treatment and bringing about quicker results. More is said about this later. The main problem, therefore, is that this method is unsuitable for recording in this way. When this method is used, the therapist has to be present in order that he may time his suggestions according to the speed of response in his patient. It is a very rare patient indeed that will respond at the same speed each time he is subjected to a hypnotic induction process.

For this reason, this method is usually only used in simple cases where only one session of treatment is required, or where reinforcement is not necessary. Therapists are therefore more likely to use approaches which can be recorded and used successfully.

Where inductions are used that are suitable for recording, certain factors must be taken into consideration. The most important of these is that people are individuals. They respond at different rates. The induction must therefore allow for this in such a way that any patient who listens to such a recording will achieve a level of hypnosis.

Such inductions therefore need a great deal of careful preparation. If, for instance, the first method discussed in this chapter were used on a recording, it is possible that the patient could suffer considerable discomfort. Such an eventuality must be avoided at all costs. A good therapist will therefore go to great lengths to make sure that his recorded inductions contain nothing which can be interpreted in such a way as to cause discomfort.

As with the above methods, there are numerous ways of inducing hypnosis on a recording. There are counting methods, trips of the imagination, metronome inductions, etc. In fact, there are too many to discuss in a book of this size.

However, all these methods, at least the good ones, have one thing in common. They are all gentle approaches. They will allow even the most distraught patients the opportunity to achieve a hypnotic level.

Regardless of this, good therapists will always satisfy themselves that the patient will respond to such an induction. They do not like to leave anything to chance. They therefore introduce the patient to hypnosis by using this induction method, and will monitor their response personally. They will also make sure that the patient becomes familiar with this induction by using the same approach at each appointment.

So far, the above has been concerned with the first stage of the induction. This is usually followed by one or two deepening processes, which will now be discussed.

Again, there are a number of deepening processes and variations available. The main purpose of the deepening process is to guide the patient to a slightly deeper level, and although it sounds rather technical, it is simply a device which is used to help you settle down and become a little more relaxed.

The simplest form of deepening process, and one of the most effective, is a period of about one minute of complete silence. This allows the patient time to adjust to the new condition and feel more relaxed. The period of silence is usually followed by a very short deepener, which acts as a bridge between the induction and the treatment.

This second deepener may simply involve the therapist counting slowly to a number of his own choice, say 5 or 10, including one or two relaxing suggestions.

Processes involving counting are very widely used, both in initial stages and deepening processes. Sometimes, the count is punctuated with suggestions, while at other times the count is used in conjunction with something else; the sound of a metronome, for instance.

Some forms of initial induction can also be used as deepening processes. One such method directs your attention to various parts of your body, and you are instructed to relax each part of the body as it is mentioned. This can be used either as the initial stage or as the deepening process. It would, however, be ridiculous for the therapist to use the same approach for both stages, and, of course, this is never done.

Imagination can be used as a deepener. You may be asked to enter a lift and descend, floor by floor, until you reach the ground floor. This has the advantage that it can be incorporated into the treatment itself as part of an imaginary analogy.

I hope that you will now have a rough idea of the kind of technique that a hypnotherapist will use to lead you into a hypnotic trance state. However, this is by no means the end of the story. Hypnosis can be induced in other ways too.

One device which is often used is called a "trigger". In the same way that a pull on the trigger of a gun brings about an instantaneous reaction, so the use of this device brings about instantaneous hypnosis.

The trigger itself may take many forms. It can be a sound, like the ting of a bell or a snap of the fingers. It can be a flash of light. Or it can be something simple, like a phrase or saying, or even just one word. The application of the trigger sets off an immediate reaction which brings about an almost instantaneous trance condition.

In order for a trigger to be successful, the patient must be no stranger to hypnosis. It would therefore not be used on your first encounter with hypnosis. There needs to be a willingness on your part to enter the trance state, and in order to achieve this it is important that you understand certain things about triggers.

The thought that often crosses the mind of people who are offered the use of a trigger is that there is a possibility that one may encounter that same trigger outside the hypnotic situation. Suppose, for instance, that your trigger was a phrase. You might find that in the middle of a conversation, that that phrase is used. Does it mean that at that point you would immediately go into a trance? The answer to that is quite simply "NO". Your trigger is given to you under hypnosis, and it is accompanied by suggestions which are designed to protect you from such eventualities. The trigger will only work when you *intend* to enter a trance state, and at no other time. Without that intention the trigger will not work, even if the therapist himself gives it to you. This is true, even if you give yourself the trigger without that intention. In other words, there is no way that you can be hypnotised accidentally.

There is, of course, individual variation in response to triggers. While some people can accept and respond to a trigger quickly and easily, others experience some difficulty. This does not mean that they cannot respond. It simply means that they lack confidence in their own ability to respond. The success comes with practice.

There are learning processes involved in hypnosis. Some people have a natural ability to respond, while others have to learn. If one fails to be hypnotised at the first attempt, it is not an indication that they cannot be hypnotised. There will be a reason for it. Perhaps the strangeness of the initial encounter was too much for them, and held them back. If so, the second attempt would be better because they now have an idea of the procedure, and realise that there is nothing to fear. Unless you are unable to maintain your concentration for more than a sentence or two, you *CAN* be hypnotised. It is simply a question of the degree to which you can co-operate with the suggestions.

6

What form does the treatment take?

If one were to ask: "What would worry you most about visiting a hypnotherapist? Is it the hypnosis, or the treatment?" In most cases, the answer would be "The hypnosis". This, however, would be the wrong answer, because the difficulties lie not in the hypnosis, but in what happens to you while you are hypnotised.

Hypnosis is simply a tool. It is the way that tool is used that is important. If you go into any household, you will find, somewhere, a screwdriver. It does not follow that the owner of the screwdriver can do every job that this tool can be used for. The owner may be capable of using the screwdriver to drive a woodscrew into a piece of carpentry, but not to use it, for instance, on a piece of electrical equipment. The effectiveness of the tool is only as good as the competence and the expertise of the user will allow.

Tools are quite often associated with trades, but some tools, like the screwdriver, are common to several trades. The craftsmen, however, use those tools only as their trade dictates. They use them in order to display their expertise effectively.

Hypnosis is just like that. It is a tool which has several applications. It can be used in many ways. A stage hypnotist, for instance, will use it to provide entertainment for an audience. A dentist will use it to make dental treatment more comfortable for the patient, and thus make his own job easier. A hypnotherapist will use it to bring about a cure for a vast range of problems, some of which are discussed here.

However, possession of the tool does not make a good craftsman. This is why the treatment is more important than the hypnosis. A qualified electrician who tries to do some carpentry will not be as good as a qualified carpenter. In the same way, a good stage hypnotist is not necessarily as good as a hypnotherapist or a dentist. The field of stage hypnosis is as far removed from hypnotherapy as it is from nuclear physics. Only the tool of hypnosis is common to both.

Once that tool has been used, the patient is ready for treatment. This is where the therapist goes to work.

For many people, the word "treatment" has a clinical ring to it. It suggests discomfort, sterilised instruments, and depersonalisation. When this word is used in connection with hypnotherapy, none of these things are involved. You are extremely comfortable. No instruments are used. But most important of all is the fact that you are treated as an individual.

The first thing that happens when you visit a hypnotherapist is that you both sit down and discuss your problem. It is important that the therapist can understand your problem *as you experience it.* Two people can suffer from the same problem, but their personal experience of it can be very different. The therapist recognises this and attaches great importance to it.

Also, at this initial consultation, the therapist will take the opportunity to explain his procedures to you and answer any questions you may have.

It is during this initial consultation that you will begin to form an opinion of your therapist. At the end of this period you should feel that here is someone who understands your problem, is concerned about it, and is prepared to do something about it. You will also find that he is very open about it and will take the time to explain things to you.

Depending upon the arrangements that you make, your introduction to hypnosis will take place there and then, or an appointment will be made for some later date. It is not unusual, at this time, for the patient to feel nervous or apprehensive about what is going to happen. This is a very natural reaction. However, you will find that your therapist will soon put you at ease, and your introduction to hypnosis should be very pleasant and enjoyable.

Once the trance state has been induced, treatment can begin. It is here that the full range of techniques can come into play, and once again, there are many techniques to choose from.

One has to remember here that one is dealing with the subconscious mind. One cannot deal with this in the same way that one deals with the conscious mind. Speaking to a subconscious mind is like talking to a very young child. One speaks slowly and deliberately and uses much repetition. One also speaks in language that can be clearly understood. In this way the point goes home and the subconscious is influenced.

It is possible to deal with some conditions simply by using direct suggestions. Smoking and slimming are dealt with in this way, as are some of the other conditions where habits are involved. Usually, this is accompanied by suggestions designed to stimulate the imagination. In this way, realisations are made, goals are clarified, and action is encouraged. In other words, it not only brings about the result, but it also makes you feel good about it. In this way smokers are able to stop the habit without loss of temper or replacing it with overeating, chocolates, sweets, chewing gum, or whatever.

It may seem strange to think that the spoken word can bring about such powerful results, which is how it seems to the patient. What in fact happens is that the spoken words stimulate the imagination, which is the really powerful force at work here. It is the imagination which transforms the spoken word into a physical response. If, for instance, it is suggested that your arm is so light that it will float into the air, then your arm will in fact float into the air. If it is suggested that your arm has heavy straps around it which are securing it down to the place where it rests, then you will be unable to move that arm, and so on. In each of these cases, the suggestion is being transformed into something physical simply through the use of the imagination.

If this process is used properly, it can be used to clear up nervous rashes, eczema, psoriasis, asthma, and many other conditions of this nature. The suggestion fires the imagination into setting into motion a physical response which will completely clear up conditions of this kind.

The list of conditions which can be treated in this way is almost endless. It ranges from smoking and slimming, to anxiety states, tension and depression, to habits like nail-biting and bed-wetting, to sports performance and driving ability, to stammering and blushing, and even as far as migraines, phobias, and hysterical paralysis.

These are just a few of the conditions which can be treated in this way. There are, of course, many more. But at the same time, one should not run away with the idea that this is the panacea for ALL ills. It does have its limitations. For instance, it will not repair a decayed tooth, or mend a broken leg (although it can speed up the healing process). Recognising this, it is always advisable for you to telephone your therapist to ask whether or not your condition can be catered for in his repertoire.

The power of suggestion can also be used for demonstration purposes. Let us suppose that you have agoraphobia; a fear of open spaces. You find that each time you go out of the house you are stricken with panic. The therapist can give you a weapon to use against these panics, so that whenever you feel the panic coming on, you can take it away yourself. If you are simply told about it, there is a possibility that you will not use it because of a fear that it might not work. By using the appropriate suggestions it is possible to demonstrate its effectiveness to the patient in such a way that they know it works. Each time the therapist tries to induce panic, the patient outwits him by taking it away. Because of this, the patient is not even mildly disturbed by the experience, and they can use the weapon confidently in their every-day lives.

From this it can be seen that there is more than one way to use the power of suggestion. It is suggestion, however, that lies behind all of the techniques used by the hypnotherapist. It is through suggestion that one can gain access to the memory bank contained in the subconscious. Under these circumstances, this access is almost unlimited. The technique used to do this is called "regression", and a separate chapter has been set aside to discuss this fascinating aspect of hypnotherapy.

Access to memory is a very important facility because very often it is the key to the whole problem. It is through this access that the cause of the problem can be uncovered. It can, for instance, indicate the nature of the problem; whether a particular event in your life lies behind your present condition, or whether a habit has developed over the years, or even whether there is some physical reason for the condition. Simple logic states that if your entire life history is recorded in your subconscious mind, then your subconscious mind will also know what steps it has taken, perhaps wrongly, in order to bring about the present state of affairs. Once this information is known, then the therapist knows how to proceed more effectively.

It should not be assumed from this that all treatments involve regression. Sometimes the same information can be obtained by other means, as the following example shows.

Let us take the case of paralysis. Paralysis can be the result of physical "accident", such as the contraction of polio, or some such disease, or perhaps an actual accident where, for instance, the nerves have been severed. It can also, however, be the result of a psychological accident, a reaction to some stressful event. In this case, there is no physical basis for the paralysis. Because of the shock of the event, the brain has decided to immobilise part of the body.

The origins of the paralysis are therefore completely different, while outwardly they appear to be the same. The physical symptoms are the same in both cases – the patient simply cannot move.

Obviously, in order to bring about an effective cure for the paralysis, the cause must be known. In some cases this is easy to do, while in others it is difficult to establish whether the cause is physical or psychological. In these cases, the power of hypnotic suggestion can be used to make this distinction. If the cause is physical, then it is physically impossible for the patient to move, regardless of the suggestions that are given. If, however, the cause is psychological, then there is nothing physical to prevent movement. In this instance, movement will occur under hypnosis.

From this it can be seen that suggestions are useful not only in treatment, but in diagnosis as well. The hypnotherapist is able to make sure that the treatment is appropriate for the individual needs of the patient through this contact with the subconscious mind.

Occasionally, it is necessary for the patient to take a good look at himself and face the problem squarely. The prospect of having to do this is often a disturbing thought. This can, however, be made much easier with the use of hypnosis. Under hypnosis, the patient is shown how to do this while also being given suggestions that are constructive and helpful as regards coping with this situation.

The purpose of this approach is to clarify a situation which may have got out of hand and reached a point where the patient is confused enough to be unable to think properly.

From this, you can see that the hypnotherapist has several

techniques at his command. There are, of course, more, but enough have been given here to give you an idea of the kind of thing that can be done with this unique treatment. Let us therefore conclude this chapter with an actual case history of a young housewife who suffered with eczema.

Christine was a young housewife in her early thirties, who suffered with eczema on the face, neck and arms. It had been on the neck and arms since about the age of three, but had moved to her face in her early twenties. Quite naturally, she found this embarrassing.

She had seen several specialists, and had had hydrocortisone treatment, acupuncture, steroids and anti-hystamines. None of these had worked for her.

Under hypnosis it was revealed that there were two major events in her life which had caused her eczema; one at the age of three and another at the age of fifteen. She was then regressed to those ages.

The stories she told seemed to have little bearing on eczema as a condition. There was nothing about infection or exposure to any other case of eczema. Instead there were two stories about family trouble, in which she found herself in an impossible position where she was asked to choose between her parents, and this at the age of three.

In both these episodes, the feeling of confusion and insecurity were very evident, and it was in fact this which had caused the eczema. A programme of treatment was devised to treat the eczema and build up her confidence. This programme combined the use of the imagination with direct suggestions. The improvements were immediate. After one week the rash was drying up. Two weeks later, she was able to wear clothes that had previously irritated her condition, and her face had visibly improved. After another two weeks, the eczema had completely gone.

To a large extent, this case is typical. A combination

of techniques are used, both to establish the cause and to treat the cause and the symptoms. At all times, nothing but the human voice is used. If this is used correctly, the patient's own imagination and determination does the rest.

7

What is regression?

One of the most powerful and impressive techniques used in hypnotherapy is that of regression. It is also one of the more controversial techniques.

Usually, when most people think of regression in connection with hypnosis, they think in terms of the more dramatic instances where people seemingly relive a previous existence, sometimes going back centuries. Such events have taken place under hypnosis. If you believe in reincarnation, then such events are fine. They will tend to support your beliefs. However, if you do not believe in this, then such events are troublesome.

It is not intended here to enter into a discussion of these weird occurrences, mainly because they are of no therapeutic value, except in extreme cases. Suffice it to say that no-one really knows what happens in these instances.

Regression is, however, used a lot in hypnotherapy. But it confines itself to what goes on in this life. In order to understand this better, we need to refer back to our model.

Let us assume that you have a problem, a phobia for instance. At some time in your life you were subjected to extraordinary stress, and this left you with an unreasonable fear of some sort. Let us also assume that you have no idea of what that event was. We can now look at our model to see what has happened.

In order for our bodies to function at all, we need memory in order to know how to do it. We could not take a breath unless we remember how we took the last breath. It therefore follows that at birth, and perhaps a little before birth, we possess a working memory.

From our model, we see that the memory is contained in the subconscious mind. Let us now assume that this memory has almost unlimited capacity. This would mean that every event that we have experienced in our lives is recorded somewhere in that subconscious memory bank. Therefore, the event that led to your phobia is also recorded there. Also recorded there is your reaction to that event, and by using this information, the subconscious mind perpetuates the fear.

We also know from our model that the conscious mind has access to that memory, but that the subconscious mind also places limitations on that access. In other words, the subconscious mind dictates just what you can, or cannot, remember. If you cannot remember the event that led to the phobia, it simply means that the subconscious is barring the way to that memory.

Looked at in this way, you can easily understand that because you cannot remember it does not mean that it is not there. It therefore becomes a question of access, and, as we have already discussed, we can gain that access through hypnosis.

Having this access is very important. By using this access, we can search that memory bank to locate the cause of the problem. Once we know the cause, then we know how to treat the condition.

Sometimes, a patient can be afraid of regression. They reason that "if something happened to me that is too painful to remember, then I don't want to face it now."

On the face of it, this is a sensible comment to make. But in practice, it is often an unfounded fear, for the following reasons. Often the cause lies in the first five years of life. If we use this as a basis, we can see that when an event occurs in the life of, say, a five-year-old child, then that child uses the reasoning of a five-year-old to evaluate that event. In denying the conscious mind access to this memory, the subconscious mind also denies access to the five-year-old reasoning that accompanies it.

If that same event happened to an adult, the outcome would be completely different for the simple reason that adult reasoning is used. The things that are important to a child are not as important to an adult. It therefore follows that, more often than not, patients who are regressed go back to events that are nowhere near as devastating as one might imagine. This is clearly shown in some of the cases quoted later in this chapter.

In order for regression to be successful, it is necessary for the subject to achieve a reasonable depth of trance. It becomes very effective when the subject is at that point where entry into unconsciousness is imminent. For this reason, it is rarely attempted at the first appointment. Subjects usually only achieve a light level on their first encounter with hypnosis.

It is, however, possible to set the stage for regression, even on that first encounter, by getting some relevant information from the subconscious, which takes the randomness out of the procedure. This is done by obtaining an "ideo-motor response", usually referred to as an I.M.R. This rather grand title simply means that the subconscious is given the opportunity to communicate through a part of the body, usually a finger.

In simple language, what happens is this. While the patient is in the trance state, suggestions are given which centre the attention of the subconscious upon the chosen part of the body, the finger for instance. The finger then becomes a direct channel for communication. The subconscious can then be asked questions about itself. It will reply to those questions by, for instance, making the finger twitch if the answer is "yes". This twitch is the I.M.R.

During this process, the conscious mind does not participate. It merely observes. This results in some patients being aware of the responses, while others are not. Much depends upon the violence of the twitch. Sometimes, the finger twitches so strongly that the whole arm moves with it. In such cases, the patients are very aware of the responses. In other cases, the twitch is barely perceptible, in which case the patient is less likely to be aware of the response.

By using this technique, the therapist can establish many things. If you think of your problem as being a trick that your brain has played on you, then the I.M.R. can be used to find out what that trick was. It can be used to establish whether the condition is physical or psychological. But its importance as far as this discussion is concerned is that it can be used to establish the time at which relevant events occurred. This, of course, means that the patient can be regressed to specific times and events, rather than aimlessly wandering through the past to find something that may be of relevance. It is therefore a time-saver, as well as a good indicator.

Armed with the I.M.R. information, the therapist can now proceed, if necessary, with the regression, having specific aims in mind. When this happens, the subject is guided into a much deeper level of hypnosis, where the subconscious is directed to unearth the information that is required.

This is one of the occasions when the subject speaks under hypnosis, describing what they see, and answering questions about it. Here again, the experience varies. For some people, it is like watching a film. They see it clearly, but are able to remain detached from it, thus diminishing their emotional involvement. Others actually relive the experience. It is as though they are actually there again. This, of course, means that because it is so real to them, they fully express their emotions.

The therapist, of course, is directing affairs, and is in full command of the situation. This enables him to make sure that the subject is not made too uncomfortable by the experience. It also enables him to take steps to ensure that on awakening, the subject is not in any state of distress, and feels calm, relaxed, and relieved.

The use of regression in hypnotherapy is probably best understood by considering a few actual case histories. The transcripts that follow demonstrate various points about regression. To protect the confidentiality of the actual patients, no names are given.

The first case shows how the cause of a condition can sometimes be blatantly obvious. Mr A. was a gentleman who suffered with a severe stammer. He had stammered for as long as he could remember. He held a position of considerable responsibility and was naturally worried about the image he was projecting. The I.M.R. process indicated the age of five as being relevant. The following is a transcript of part of the session at which he was regressed.

"Where are you now?"
". . . At home."
"And how old are you?"
"I'm five."
"And what are you doing?"
". . . I'm worried."
"What are you worried about?"
". . . I've dropped a knife . . . can't find it."
"Which room are you in?"
"The kitchen . . . I've dropped the knife."
"Why can't you find it?"
"It's rolled under something."
"Does this worry you?"
"Yes . . . Want to find it."
"What is happening now?"
"My father has come into the kitchen."
"What is he doing?"

"Asked me what I had dropped."

"Was he concerned?"

"No . . . He was demanding an explanation . . . very aggressive . . . sounded angry."

"So what happens?"

". . . Can't get the words out."

"So what did you say?"

"A kn–n–n–nife."

"So you stumbled over your words?"

"Yes . . . Couldn't say it."

"Why did you do this? Were you afraid?"

"Yes . . . worried."

"Because you were afraid of your father?"

"Yes."

"What did your father do then?"

"He made me sit in a chair and practice words."

"Why did he do that?"

"He didn't want me to stammer."

"So he made you practice words?"

"Yes."

"How did he do it?"

"He said a word and I had to repeat it after him."

"How long did this take?"

"About an hour each day."

"Each day?"

"A long time . . . months."

"Did you find that you stammered more as time went on?"

"Yes."

"And the more you stammered, the more you had to practice?"

"Yes."

"How did your father react to this?"

"He got more aggressive . . . and more angry."

"Why do you think this was?"

"I think he felt ashamed of me."

It takes very little imagination to see from this the cause of
his stammer. The father, through his own stupidity, had
meticulously taught his son to stammer.

Not all cases are this obvious. Mr B. also suffered with
a severe stammer. His I.M.R. also gave the age of five. But
this is what happened in this case:

"Where are you now?"

"In the street."

"How old are you?"

"Five."

"What are you doing?"

"Playing with friends."

"What game are you playing?"

"There's a sort of grating outside this shop . . . We're
hitting it with a brick."

"Why are you doing that?"

"Don't know . . . Just playing."

"What happened then?"

"We broke it . . . The grating."

"And then what?"

"Ran . . . Ran home."

"Did you get away with it?"

"No."

"Why? What happened?"

"Another boy . . . a friend . . . came along and fell in the
hole . . . Tripped up and his leg went in."

"Was he hurt?"

"Yes . . . Broke his leg."

"What happened then?"

"His Mum came to our house and told my Mum off."

"What did your Mum do?"

"She told me off . . . and gave me a clip round the ear."

"Was that the end of it?"

"No. Mum told Dad . . . when he came home."

"And what did he do?"

"Same as Mum."
"Another clip round the ear?"
"Yes."
"How did you feel then?"
"Frightened."
"Why?"
"In case my friend didn't get better."
"But he did, didn't he?"
"Yes."

As you read this account you were probably wondering what possible connection it could have with stammering. There is no mention of speech at all. However, further investigation showed that Mr B. suffered severe guilt feelings as a result of his friend's broken leg, and he did, in fact, express this by copying the stammer from another acquaintance. This stammer had developed over the years until it became habitual.

An interesting point about stammerers is that under hypnosis they speak clearly and well, with no sign of an impediment. This fact was made use of with both these cases. Recordings were made of their own voices speaking under hypnosis, in which they used words which were problematical to them. The recordings were played back to them after the sessions, and used during later sessions of hypnosis. These procedures, together with rationalising suggestions brought about immediate improvements in their speech.

Regressions can sometimes be amusing, as well as informative, as the following case shows.

Mr C. was a patient who had a fear of crashing while flying. As he had to travel abroad as part of his job several times a year, this was a serious problem for him. His I.M.R. indicated two ages of importance, but here, we will only be concerned with one of them.

"Where are you?"

"I'm in hospital."

"How old are you?"

"I'm three."

"Why are you in hospital?"

"I'm going to have an operation on my eye."

"What's wrong with your eye? Do you know?"

"It keeps going in the corner."

"I see. What are you doing now?"

"I'm underneath the bed."

"Underneath the bed?"

"Yes."

"Why are you there?"

"I'm playing."

"What are you playing?"

"I'm playing with an aeroplane that somebody has given me as a present for going into hospital."

"You'll get into trouble for that won't you?"

"Yes."

"O.K. Who caught you?"

"One of the nurses."

"What did she do?"

"Told me off and took it away."

This punishment seemed a little drastic for so small a crime, and so he was questioned more closely about this incident. It transpired that when he was taken into the hospital and safely installed in his bed, he decided to play with the toy aeroplane. Unfortunately, it had been placed in his bedside locker. He couldn't reach it, so he got out of bed. Having retrieved the toy from the locker, he then found that he could not climb back into bed as it was too high. He therefore decided to play on the floor. But, as with all children of that age, the game spread out as he got more involved in it. This resulted in him zooming up and down the ward, under everybody else's beds, making loud aeroplane noises.

However, although this conjures up some amusing pictures of the situation, the tragedy was that the operation was a failure. Coupled with this was the fact that he never saw that toy again.

Years later, another event took place in which he was playing football in a field next to an aerodrome. As they played, bombers were taking off and landing. The noise from the aircraft was deafening, to the extent that the ground vibrated, his head throbbed, and he couldn't hear properly for a few days afterwards.

In his mind, he had then made an association between aeroplanes and the loss of one of the senses. He then rationalised that the only way this could happen was for the aeroplane to crash. Thus the fear developed.

During the following week, he thought about the regression and realised himself that his fears were unfounded. There followed one more session of treatment, after which he was able to fly comfortably, without that feeling of impending doom.

Sometimes, when a regression is attempted, the subconscious tries to put up a barrier. Quite often, this barrier can be overcome with a little persuasion. When this happens, it takes a little time for the picture to form before it becomes clear. This is illustrated in the following example.

"Where are you now Claire?"
Silence.
"What place can you see?"
Silence.
"Can you describe to me what you can see?"
"Nothing."
"Nothing at all?"
Silence.
"Do you not get even a small picture? A very quick glimpse of something?"

". . . Car."

"What sort of car is it? Do you know?"

". . . Mini."

"What colour is it?"

". . . Blue."

"What is it doing?"

". . . Travelling."

"Is it going fast?"

"No."

"Who is in the car?"

"Mum, Dad, and my brother."

From this point on, the picture gradually emerged until it became clear, and a full account could be given.

Occasionally, a regression attempt will fail, but this does not mean that all is lost. Hypnotherapy is a very versatile discipline, and there are procedures which can be used which will achieve the same end result. Regression, however, has the advantage that it is very direct, and therefore saves time.

The above examples are very typical of the kind of thing that happens with regression. Occasionally, however, one comes across a horrific event; an event too painful to remember. Here, the versatility of the discipline comes into play. While it is important that the information be obtained, the therapist recognises that remembering such an event may be detrimental to the treatment at that particular time. He can therefore give suggestions to the effect that the patient will have no recollection of the session on awakening. They will simply feel that they went to sleep and missed it altogether. The therapist, on the other hand, now knows the story. He now knows what he is dealing with. He can therefore take the necessary steps to overcome the problem.

Regression can be used in many ways. Here, we have mainly dealt with the therapeutic aspect. There are, however, other situations in which a memory search is useful.

As an illustration of this, consider a situation where an item of value has been lost; perhaps something of sentimental value. Searching the subconscious memory with regression has often resulted in the location of the lost item, much to the satisfaction of its owner.

From the above, it is hoped that the value of regression can be seen. Its directness and accuracy make it invaluable as a tool for use in therapy. It is by far the best agent in finding the key to the mystery of the patient's problems.

8

Anxiety? Tension? Depression?

Anxiety is the factor that lies behind most of the problems in which the mind plays a part. It is the main product of stress, and can lead to serious problems if the conditions are appropriate.

Anxiety can be described as a state of apprehension or uneasiness, which is related to fear. The cause of the anxiety can be something specific, such as a vicious animal, or it can be something vague, like an idea that something might happen.

From this simple state of anxiety, the situation can develop in several directions. It can, for instance, develop into a continual feeling of dread, accompanied by tension, palpitation, sweating and nausea. It can also develop into depression, phobias, obsessions, or hysteria. It can even be the reason why someone smokes. In short, it lies behind most of the conditions which can be treated with hypnotherapy.

Wherever anxiety is involved, the first thing to go is the ability to remain calm and relaxed. When the anxiety is strong enough, relaxation becomes impossible, and a state of tension prevails. This is commonly experienced as a "knotted up" feeling in the stomach, which spreads over the entire body. This is often accompanied by feelings of not knowing what to do; as though looking for something but not knowing what one is looking for. The overall feeling is one of desperation and panic. There are obviously degrees to which this can be experienced, but whatever the degree, it is unpleasant.

Anxiety can also lead to depression. This may, or may not, be accompanied by tension. Again, this is unpleasant to experience. All interest in life reaches a very low ebb. One becomes lethargic and apathetic. There seems to be no purpose to anything. When work is done, it is done mechanically, with no interest or enthusiasm. And so it goes on.

Often, people who suffer from this type of problem are taking some type of antidepressant medication. This often leads to its own problems, because many of the antidepressant drugs are addictive. Consequently, a patient taking this medication will find that the depression goes, but then finds that they have become dependent upon the drug. The depression therefore returns, but it is now aggravated by the fact that the drug is also necessary. This second depression thus becomes worse than the original problem.

The next step in this progression is usually a trip to the psychiatrist, the psychologist, the neurologist, or some other specialist in the field. Often, the patient is shunted from one specialist to another. Each one will conduct his own tests and offer his own brand of treatment. In some cases this is successful, but in many cases it is not.

Most of the patients who come to a hypnotherapist with this type of problem have been through this mill. Many of these have also undergone electro-convulsive shock treatment (E.C.T.), but to no avail. While E.C.T. is fairly widely used, and enjoys a reasonable success rate, this is of little comfort to those for whom it does not work.

So let us now look at the way in which hypnotherapy can be of use with this type of problem.

Once again, the key thought is that people are individuals. Although they may be suffering from anxiety, tension and/or depression, they experience this in very individual ways. Whereas a headache, for instance, can be experienced in several ways (i.e. a sharp, stabbing pain, or a dull throbbing pain), so too there is variation in the experience of anxiety, tension and depression.

At your initial consultation, the therapist will be interested in knowing what your personal experience is, in order that he may approach it in the right way. He will also ask you questions about your life, both past and present. All this is necessary in order that the therapist can understand your problem fully, and how it affects you as an individual. Where it is relevant, this sometimes means divulging very personal information. However, therapists are bound by strict rules of confidentiality. Any information you give is kept strictly between you and your therapist. Your therapist cannot even discuss your case with another specialist unless he has your written permission to do so.

It is at this initial consultation that the therapist must decide upon the viability of taking the case on. In view of the above, this may seem a strange thing to say, but there is one circumstance where it would be pointless to take the case on.

Occasionally, one comes across a case where the patient finds that by suffering in this way they get a lot of attention from those around them. Usually this is found amongst those who typically lead a lonely kind of existence. Consequently, they develop a fear that if they get better, then they will lose that attention, and will once again have to fend for themselves. In other words, the benefits from being ill outweigh the benefits from being well. Once this decision has been made, then it cannot be said that the patient really wants to get better, or is prepared to do something about it.

Under these circumstances, there is no point in attempting treatment, since that treatment would not be in harmony with the patient's wishes. The patient would therefore reject any suggestions leading them to good health, and the treatment would be guaranteed to fail. However, where these circumstances do not prevail, treatment can happily proceed.

Also, at this initial consultation, the therapist must decide on the treatment he will use. In order to do this, his line of questioning will be aimed at finding out the cause of the problem. Sometimes the cause is obvious, such as the depression following a divorce, the birth of a child, a bereavement, etc. This enables a straightforward approach to be used. If the cause is not clear, then the therapist will consider the use of the I.M.R. and regression.

Following this consultation, the stage is set for treatment to begin. Usually, the first stage is for the patient to be given some relaxation therapy. This helps to combat the anxiety. It also serves as a good introduction to hypnosis, because it is not necessary for the patient to achieve any great depth of trance for the benefits to be felt.

During this session, the therapist will ensure that the patient is responding properly. Not only will he look for the signs that are displayed in hypnosis, but he will also conduct a test, which will not only confirm this but will also put the patient's mind at rest. It could be suggested, for instance, that an arm has been strapped down so that it cannot be moved. If the patient finds he cannot move that arm, even though there is nothing there, then the patient also knows that something has happened.

Depending on the situation, suggestions may be given that are aimed specifically at the condition being treated.

In subsequent sessions, the treatment really gets to grips with the problem. One of the things that must be considered is the fact that the mind can make the condition habitual. Steps must therefore be taken to ensure that any such habit is broken. The situation that brought the condition about must also be rationalised.

It therefore follows that the phase of treatment following the introduction to hypnosis would be one of investigation. It is during this phase that the therapist discovers what caused the condition in the first place. If the condition was the result of a specific event, then that event is discovered at this time. It is also discovered whether that event is still of relevance to the patient. Also ascertained is whether or not the condition is the result of a habitual response, whether there is a physical reason for the condition to prevail, and whether or not the patient's emotions are involved, such as the suppression of feelings of guilt over an event which occurred many years ago.

It is during this phase of treatment that the situation really becomes clear. It is also during this phase of treatment that the relationship between patient and therapist is of vital importance. The patient must be assured that whatever happens between the patient and therapist is kept strictly confidential. It may be that the condition results from something that the patient would not want others to know. It is therefore essential that the patient feels able to trust his therapist.

Having gained this information, the therapist is now in a position to enter the third phase of the treatment. This third phase of treatment concerns dealing with the cause of the problem, whatever it may be. This can involve the rationalisation of past events, the breaking of habits, the freeing of suppressed emotions, and so on. It can take many forms. On occasion, it is possible for the therapist to begin this phase at the same time as the investigative process finishes, depending, of course, on the gravity of the situation.

One final phase of treatment is necessary. This concerns dealing with the symptoms of the condition. It is often the case that once a cause has been established and dealt with, that a condition will cease to exist. However, one must remember that a patient may have been living with that problem for a considerable number of years. Therefore, that problem has become a way of life to that patient. To be suddenly free from a condition after a lengthy period of time means that a period of adjustment to a new way of life is necessary, and with conditions of this kind help is needed in adjusting to that new way of life. So this is the function of that fourth phase of treatment. This is the part where the patient is helped to adjust to a life that is free of those irritating symptoms that have been displayed in the past.

Having passed through these four phases of treatment, the patient is usually over the problem and is able to carry out a more normal way of life. However, particularly in cases where long periods of suffering are concerned, a patient will take time to adjust, and although they are able to carry out a normal way of life, they like to feel that they have a lifeline available to them. Usually this is easily accomplished, for the simple reason that during the course of the treatment, the relationship that builds between patient and therapist is one of friendship. The patient therefore feels that the therapist is approachable and will quite often simply telephone the therapist, just for a talk, or perhaps call in at the consulting rooms for a chat, just to straighten their own thoughts and seek advice perhaps. This may result in one or two more sessions of treatment, but only if absolutely necessary. More often it is simply a chat, concerned with how that patient has fared, and develops into a talk between friends. The important thing, however, is that by the time this stage has been reached, the problem has been overcome.

9

Phobias?

Fear is something that most people have experienced at some time in their lives. It may have been a moment of panic or, maybe a prolonged session of fear. Usually, this is the result of a confrontation with a dangerous situation, a situation which arouses very strong feelings in that person – the feeling that we call "fear".

For most people the experience of fear has a solid foundation. A woman alone in a house at night with a prowler going around the outside of the house feels panic and fear. Until such time as that situation is resolved, and even beyond that point, fear remains. Conversely, there is the momentary experience of fear. As you step out into the road and see a car coming with only a split second in which to retreat, if you are to avoid an accident, then during that time you feel panic.

With instances of this kind the danger is very real. Phobias, on the other hand, are something different. With a phobia, a person experiences fear even in the absence of a real danger. For example, a person with a fear of heights will experience a dreadful panic whenever at any height above ground level. It may be that in that situation, the person is in no danger of any kind. They may be perfectly safe and very secure, but the fact that they are high above the ground will instil a dreadful fear in that person, feelings of uncontrollable panic and terror. It is this kind of fear that the word "phobia" refers to.

Phobias can be related to many, many things, there is the fear of heights mentioned above, the fear of open spaces, the fear of confined spaces, the fear of darkness, a fear of thunder and lightning, and many, many others. Each one of these fears is a very disturbing thing to experience, because with each one of these cases the patient has feelings of blind te: ror and panic.

From this it can be seen that a phobia is a very disturbing thing to live with. It is therefore not uncommon to find that patients who suffer with phobias also suffer with depression, because of the disturbing influence it has upon their lives, to the extent that it prevents them conducting their lives in a normal way. Accompanying the fear, are feelings of tension and intense anxiety. Their lives are lived under complete threat. Sometimes, with a fear of heights for instance, it is possible to avoid the situation as much as possible. A person suffering with this kind of phobia will therefore go to great lengths to avoid being at any height above ground level. On the other hand, a person with a fear of thunder and lightning is not in a position to avoid a thunder-storm. Thunder-storms arrive at the whim of nature. They therefore live their lives waiting for the next thunder-storm. Usually people with such phobias take intense interest in weather forecasts. Some of them even 'phone weather stations each day to try to assess whether or not there will be a storm that day. With this situation, the person lives in perpetual fear because there is no way they can avoid that storm in the way that a person with a fear of heights can avoid climbing to heights.

Since phobias are anxiety-based, the treatment for this condition follows the same procedures that were discussed in chapter eight, the same four phases of treatment have to be gone through. Of course, much emphasis in this case is placed on the investigative phase, in establishing where the fear arose, how it began. The I.M.R. and regression techniques are therefore often used with this kind of condition.

Whereas the four phases mentioned above are gone through, there are other additions to this treatment for this particular condition.

It has to be remembered that the condition will have had a very definite effect on the patient's way of life. If, for instance, they have avoided heights for many years, then find they have the ability to go to a height and feel comfortable, the first occasion will be a very strange and perhaps harrowing experience, and before actually experiencing it, they will feel a great deal of apprehension and nervousness. Here again, hypnotherapy can help, because the therapist can prepare the patient for this event. He can make them experience it in their imagination before experiencing it in reality. The hypnotherapist can get the patient to imagine as though it were real, facing whatever it is that is the object of fear, under hypnosis. It is at this time that the therapist arms the patient with a defensive weapon. The patient is shown a technique, whereby they can control the strong feelings of apprehension and nervousness that are naturally bound to occur. Under hypnosis, the patient will go to a great height, controlling emotions and feelings throughout the entire experience. The feelings that are experienced under hypnosis are real. If the hypnotist suggests that a feeling of panic is rising up within that person, then that patient will actually experience the panic. But then the therapist will get the patient to use the weapon to take away that feeling of panic, and control it.

This technique is extremely effective. Many patients who have learnt this technique have found the experience of facing up to their object of fear in reality a far easier thing to do, knowing that they have a weapon that they can use against that object of fear. This enables them to become more confident, which is essential because one of the things which is lost when one suffers with a phobia is confidence.

When a patient encounters an object of fear and is able to deal with it successfully, then this experience on its own is a therapy in itself, because once they know that they can face that situation successfully, then this is something positive upon which to build. The therapist, therefore, is not only concerned with treating the condition, but is also concerned with getting the patient, in a practical sense, to be able to go through an experience that hitherto had been terrifying for that patient.

Of course, some phobic states are more common than others. It is comparatively rare to find someone with a fear of trees, while on the other hand it is very common to find a fear of open spaces. This condition is called "agoraphobia". It is a condition which is commonly found among young housewives who have a child. Often it results from the fact that when the child is born, the housewife embarks upon a five year period of devotion to that child. Five years with more time spent at home, within the confines of those four walls, simply looking after the new arrival. When that five years is over, the child is at school age, and the mother then tries to settle back to a normal way of living, but she finds that during that five years the world has changed. Traffic conditions are more intense. She no longer has the protection of those four walls. She feels exposed. She no longer feels safe. In this way the seeds of agoraphobia are implanted, and this can reach enormous proportions until that young mother finds that she is unable to go outside her home without feeling panic and terror.

This condition, however, is not confined to young mothers. Many other people also suffer from agoraphobia. For these people too, the experience is equally disturbing. Whereas the cause may be different, the experience is the same.

When it comes to treatment, agoraphobia is a special case, as it seems to be one of the easier conditions to be treated through hypnotherapy. One of the reasons for this may be that it is very difficult for one to conduct any kind of life without going outside the four walls of the home.

Therefore the patient is forced to face that fear, and thus perhaps experience it more often than someone with, say, a fear of heights. This in turn would make it easier for the agoraphobic to put themselves in a position where they have to face that fear. Whereas someone with a fear of heights is easily able, in most cases, to avoid heights, an agoraphobic finds it very difficult to avoid open spaces. This therefore means that as treatment continues, they are likely to confront their fears more quickly and more often than with many of the other phobias. As they do this and achieve success, then they learn from this very quickly, with the result, of course, that success also comes more easily and quickly than with most other phobias.

Perhaps at this point it might be a good idea to quote a case concerning agoraphobia, which will demonstrate the effectiveness of this treatment.

The patient was a housewife who had suffered with agoraphobia for sixteen years. She had been to various medical practitioners to get treatment and each one of these had failed. She had seen psychiatrists, again with no result. At the time of coming for treatment using hypnotherapy, she was taking four drugs, which had been prescribed for her. At her initial consultation, she was quaking in terror. She was in a cold sweat and was visibly trembling. This was the result of the journey that she had had to make in order to come for treatment.

The case was accepted and treatment began. Within a period of approximately four weeks, that patient was going on expeditions around the local countryside, and enjoying it. A few weeks later, she was no longer taking the medications that had been prescribed for her, and she was living a new life, appreciating and enjoying that new life.

Approximately eighteen months have passed since she began treatment to the time of writing this account. During that time she has learnt to live a very normal life. In no way does she experience any of the symptoms of agoraphobia, and at this point, her life has returned to normality.

For those of you reading this who suffer with agoraphobia, you may find this hard to believe. Many sufferers of this condition have been told that this is a condition they must learn to live with, and learn to cope with. But this is just not true. The condition can be cured, as this case clearly demonstrates. This case does not stand in isolation. Many patients have received treatment for agoraphobia using hypnotherapy, and many patients have found a total relief from that terrible fear that has dominated their lives for so long.

10

Psychosomatic conditions?

A psychosomatic condition is best described as a physical complaint which has a psychological origin. These may take many forms. Some of the commonest psychosomatic conditions include such things as stomach ulcers, asthma, eczema and psoriasis. Each one of these complaints is displayed physically. In some way or other, the individual's physical health is impaired, but in each of these cases too, the condition has been brought about as a result of stress.

If one refers back to the model used in the early chapters of this book, it can be seen that the stress we perceive in the environment affects our physical being. One way of describing this is to simply say that thought itself has a chemical component. It works in the following way.

When you think a thought of any kind, your brain releases a chemical. That chemical sets off other reactions, including the familiar electrical reaction that is commonly referred to when one talks about nerve activity. Obviously, the chemicals that are released can stimulate the release of other chemicals. Certain nervous discharges will release chemicals. It therefore follows that if under stress we are releasing chemicals, we can release chemicals that are harmful to us, as well as those which can help us to cope with the stressful situation. If an acidic chemical is released in the stomach, an ulcer will ensue. Similarly, the release of other chemicals in other areas of the body can bring about skin complaints, respiratory problems, and many of the other body functions that are necessary to the smooth operation of the body can be impaired.

Since thought can produce physical change, we are therefore confronted with a whole series of conditions that can be classed as psychosomatic.

One could, at this point, enter into a philosophical discussion in which it was argued that all illnesses are psychosomatic insofar as all illnesses have a psychological component. Even with a broken leg, there is a psychological reaction to that event, and that psychological reaction can determine how quickly one recovers from such a condition. The difference is that here we are talking about the reaction to the event which produced the physical condition, rather than about a physical condition resulting from a reaction to stress.

However, it can be said that since all illnesses have a psychological component, then if that component can be treated in an appropriate way, the healing processes can be accelerated, and in practice this is found to be the case. It therefore follows that in many of the situations discussed here, some of the principles can be applied to "ordinary" illnesses insofar as the speed of recovery is concerned. The discussion, however, will centre around those conditions which are generally classed as psychosomatic.

In the preceding chapters, we have dealt with conditions of the mind in which no physical component is really relevant. In treating those conditions, a series of procedures were adopted, and, just as before, those same four procedures are again used with psychosomatic conditions. However, in this case an addition is made.

When the patient has been introduced to hypnosis, and when the treatment is under way and the patient is responding well (i.e. achieving a degree of depth in the trance), then it is possible to use a technique in which the body is encouraged to heal itself. With this technique, the suggestions given are designed to make the body react

automatically by producing chemicals which will undo the
work of those damaging chemicals which have brought
about the conditions, and which perpetuate it.

Obviously, with such a technique, one is directly influence the subconscious mind, because it is easily appreciated
that conscious control over body functions is a difficult
thing to achieve in most cases. One of the things a therapist
will find useful in doing this is to get the imagination to
work. So, when using this technique, the therapist will feed
the imagination in order that the imagination may also
influence the subconscious mind. In simple language, it is
as though the therapist is providing a blueprint for the
subconscious mind to work upon; by giving verbal suggestions, a plan of attack is outlined. The subconscious
mind, responding to this, goes about a task of reparation.

To the uninitiated, this may sound incredible. The
thought that somebody can talk to somebody else, and
simply by doing this, clear up a dreadful skin condition like
psoriasis, is inconceivable. Yet in practice, this is exactly
what happens.

In an earlier chapter it was mentioned that a therapist will
test a patient's response. He can do this in many ways. For
example, he could suggest that the patient's arm becomes so
rigid that it just will not bend. In doing this, the therapist
makes no contact of a physical nature with that patient in
any way. All he does is say the words. The patient, on the
other hand, accepts that suggestion by listening to those
words, and then he brings about a physical change, so that
the arm does become rigid to the extent that the therapist
can then pick up that arm and try to bend it with all
his strength. But that arm will not bend. The patient has
accepted that suggestion and brought about a physical
change.

Similarly, there have been several occasions where surgi-
cal operations have been carried out without the use of
anaesthetic. Instead, hypnotic suggestions were given to

deaden the area where the operation was to be carried out. In each of these cases, the operation proceeded as though the patient had been anaesthetised in the conventional manner. But also in each of these cases, what had happened was that the patient had accepted suggestions and transformed them into an actual physical change – deadening an area of the body so that surgery could take place.

If it is possible to bring about such physical changes in this way, is it therefore so unreasonable to accept that other physical changes can also be achieved in the same way? Of course not.

This technique can also be used for conditions which are not truly psychosomatic. As an example of this, there was the case of a patient who fell down the stairs. He was not badly hurt, and only suffered a few bruises. What he did not know was that he had cracked the bone in his elbow. He was completely unaware of this, and suffered no discomfort from it. A few days later, his son pointed out to him that his elbow was swollen, and so he went to see his doctor. The doctor informed him that this swelling was a "bursa", which means that some of the fluid which lubricates the elbow joint had leaked out through the crack in the bone and had caused the swelling. The patient was informed that, if he wished, he could have the bursa drained surgically, but that if he was in no pain it might be better to wait a few months to see if it would go away naturally. The patient decided not to have surgery and went to see his hypnotherapist. He was given one session of treatment in which the above technique was used, and within three days the bursa was gone.

This technique then, is very valuable and has a very wide application. In cases like the above, it is used to speed up the body's own natural healing processes. With psychosomatic conditions it is used to clear up long-standing conditions.

However, these two applications have to be kept separate, because with psychosomatic conditions, the cause is all-important. Therefore, the technique is used in conjunction with the four procedures discussed earlier. Used in this way, the condition is not only cleared up, but it *stays* cleared up.

11

Social problems?

The preceding chapters have mainly been concerned with the treatment of conditions affecting both mental and physical health. There is, however, another area in which hypnotherapy can be useful, and that is in the field of social problems.

Social problems come in many shapes and sizes, but for our purposes we will subdivide them into two broad categories: habits and learning skills.

Habits include such things as smoking, nail-biting, bed-wetting, and other things of this kind. Also included here are slimming problems, because to a large extent, over-weight is the result of "bad" eating habits.

For the vast majority of people, habits of this nature can be overcome quickly and easily through the use of hypnosis. However, some points need to be clarified here.

Reference has been made in earlier chapters to the fact that there are good and not-so-good therapists in practice. A poor therapist will give suggestions like: "Whenever you light a cigarette in the future, you will begin to cough and will be violently sick." This approach is called "aversion therapy" and is not very successful. The lack of success is largely due to the fact that you will not respond to a suggestion that you are not in favour of. The people that do respond to this type of approach are those who think: "That is the kind of suggestion I want." But such people are in a minority.

Also, when aversion therapy is used, the patient is often tempted to try out the suggestion to see if it works. They will *try* to smoke a cigarette, or bite their nails, or whatever. But in so doing, they place themselves back in the position they were in before, and the habit begins again.

So good therapists do not resort to aversion therapy techniques. Their approach is far more positive and encouraging. The suggestions they use introduce the concept that it is possible for you to break the habit that is causing you distress. Using this as a foundation, the suggestions that follow are designed to make this possibility become a reality. No suggestions of a disturbing nature are made at all.

By using this approach, it has been found that a very high rate of success can be achieved. Care must therefore be taken in choosing a therapist, and in this respect, you will find the final chapter of this book useful.

Usually, when treating a habit, it is not necessary to undertake a long course of treatment, but on occasion the habit has developed from something else that may be more serious. In this instance, other procedures may need to be used, similar to the four procedures mentioned in the earlier chapters.

The inference here is that, just as with any of the other conditions that can be treated with hypnotherapy, the individuality of the patient is important. Giving up smoking, for instance, can be very easily accomplished by some people, while others find it almost impossible. Because of this, those who can stop easily do not require treatment at all. But of those who do need treatment, there are some who will require more treatment than others. Good therapists are aware of this, and therefore make sure that a patient having difficulty has some form of back-up service and after-care available to them, as well as the extra treatment that is necessary.

At the time of writing this book, there is an increase in

the number of establishments that are opening up which offer the use of video recordings as a means of stopping smoking or losing weight. These video recordings carry a hypnotic induction, and can therefore be referred to as a form of hypnotherapy. But it is a very bad form of hypnotherapy because it takes away the individuality of the patients. Because it is a recording it is stereotyped. No consideration is given to the inividuality of the patients. Also, because it is a recording, it is assumed that there is no need for an actual therapist to be present and the patients are therefore attended to by receptionists and other unqualified personnel. The disadvantages and dangers of this are obvious and go a long way to explaining the poor results produced by such establishments.

Before leaving the subject of habits, a word needs to be said about such habits as bed-wetting, because to a large extent this is concerned with the treatment of children. Generally speaking, children are excellent subjects for hypnosis. However, a certain level of maturity needs to have been reached for hypnotherapy to be successful. This is largely a language problem in that the child may not properly understand the suggestions being given. As a general rule, a child of normal intelligence will have reached the required level of maturity at about the age of seven. Children of lesser intelligence take longer to mature and may not be able to respond to a hypnotic induction until about eleven or twelve. The parents of the child would therefore need to discuss this aspect with the therapist at the earliest opportunity.

The final topic for discussion in this section is concerned with the learning of skills, and again, this has several aspects. You may enjoy playing a particular sport and wish to improve your technique. You may be learning to play a musical instrument and wish to apply yourself to it more successfully. You may be studying a subject at college or university and wish to improve your learning ability. You may also wish to overcome the nervousness of the examination situation. You may wish to improve your memory. There are many situations that can fall within this category.

Generally speaking, the treatment for this kind of requirement involves a short course of a few sessions of therapy. Again, the individuality of the patient comes into play. If one considers the world of sport, for instance, there is a considerable variation in the requirements of the patients. If you play, say, snooker as a hobby, then you may just be interested in improving your general performance. You may wish to improve your concentration and thus play more accurate shots. If, on the other hand, you are a world champion snooker player, then your requirements are completely different. At this level, specific shots are important, the match-play situation itself is important, the way you view your opponent is important, and so on. But regardless of the level at which you play, and regardless of your personal requirements, hypnotherapy can certainly help you to improve. There are many case histories on record of world-class sportsmen (and women) who have successfully used hypnotherapy as a means of retaining their prowess or to help them get back into the game after a disaster.

Obviously, the learning situation extends to the student. One could be studying an academic subject or simply learning a skill for personal satisfaction, such as learning to play an instrument. Whatever the case may be, the laws governing the situation are the same. You wish to be able to take in knowledge, retain it, and recall it whenever necessary, and then put it into effect.

There is no reason why any of us should not be able to do this. Yet some of us encounter enormous problems when placed in this situation. Sometimes, no matter how many times you read a page of writing, it just does not seem to go in. Sometimes, it goes in but is immediately forgotten. Sometimes, it is retained but cannot be remembered at the appropriate time.

For the academic student, the examination can be a gruelling experience. The information is there, it has been well-learnt and well-understood, but once inside the examination hall, it all crumbles and becomes a jumble of meaningless nonsense. Even the questions on the paper do not seem to make sense. Eventually, all hope disappears and panic sets in.

Some, or all of these problems are commonly encountered among students and are a cause of considerable stress among those individuals. Yet all of these things can be overcome through the use of hypnotherapy, as many people can testify, whose lives have been changed as a result of this treatment.

It is hoped that by now, you, the reader, have a better understanding and a clearer picture in your mind of what hypnotherapy is all about and the kind of things it can be used for. Being armed with this information, it may be that at some time in the future you may feel that you could benefit from a course of hypnotherapy and thus be in the position where you need to find a good therapist.

Having read this far, you will be aware that reference has consistently been made throughout this book to the fact that there are good and bad therapists, and therefore that the choice of therapist is an important issue. It is for this reason that the final chapter in this book has been devoted to this very question – the choice of a good therapist.

12

How to find a good therapist

Hypnotherapy is a specialist profession. It needs to be in the hands of people who are dedicated, knowledgeable, and skilled in the techniques of hypnotherapy. A good therapist is therefore an expert, who devotes himself to full-time practice and thus has much experience upon which to draw. He will also be a member of a reputable organisation, such as the Institute of Curative Hypnotherapists or the National Council of Psychotherapists. He will also be a person who has feeling for others, and can understand their problems. In other words, he is a professional.

Unfortunately, it is a fact of life that there are more "dabblers" than professionals. It is also a regrettable fact of life that many of the hypnotherapists who work on a professional basis are not truly professional. It is also true that some of the doctors who include hypnotherapy as part of their repertoire and use it in their general practices are inadequately trained.

The consequence of this situation is that a person seeking treatment with hypnotherapy is faced with the prospect of finding a good therapist. The purpose of this chapter is to assist you to do just that, by separating the wheat from the chaff, using a process of elimination.

First of all, it should not be inferred from the above that any attempt is being made to degrade or diminish in any way the work of doctors. They do, after all, provide an invaluable service to the community. But the medical profession is a structured profession. It is geared in such a way that if a general practitioner feels that a case is beyond his scope, he will refer that case to a specialist – someone with more expertise in that particular field. In this instance, the G.P. is acknowledging his own limitations and allowing the patient to take advantage of the more advanced knowledge of the specialist. This is obviously a good thing, since the life of the patient may be involved.

However, when it comes to hypnotherapy, the medical profession as such has very few full-time specialists. The G.P. therefore has to refer patients outside the confines of established medicine or learn to use it personally.

When it comes to referrals, the doctor is often no better informed than you are unless he knows personally of a good practitioner in his area. Usually he will confess this to the patient, sometimes referring instead to a psychiatrist who may occasionally use hypnosis.

From this it can be seen that some doctors are not in a good position here. They may therefore enrol on a course in order to learn the techniques themselves. But here they find themselves in trouble, because they are already in a profession which keeps them busy for most of their waking life, working at a fast pace. The course will teach them the rudiments of hypnotherapy and they will then try to fit this in with their normal working lives. This means that they will be using hypnotherapeutic techniques very much on a part-time basis, which in turn means that it will take a very long time to accumulate enough experience to be truly effective. They will produce results, but it will be a long and laborious process.

Their only other alternative is to give up their profession in order to take up full-time hypnotherapy. A few doctors have in fact done this, with great success. It has involved a period of further instruction during which they have become acquainted with the full spectrum of the techniques of hypnotherapy. Those who had developed an authoritarian attitude towards their patients have dropped this in favour of a more humanitarian attitude. They now find that they hypnotise more people in one month than they would otherwise have treated in an entire career. In other words, they have become specialists.

Such doctors, however, are very hard to find, and even then, they are no better than any other good hypnotherapist who does not have their medical training, since it is the doctor that has adopted the techniques already being used by hypnotherapists.

The term "dabbler" also applies to stage hypnotists. In the world of entertainment there are several individuals who use hypnosis as a means of entertaining an audience. Like all performers, they achieve a reputation and their names become familiar to hoardes of people. Some of these performers feel that because they use hypnosis, they are automatically qualified to advertise themselves as therapists, even though they have little or no training in this field, while at the same time being reluctant to give up the stage profession.

The stage hypnotist who wishes to call himself a hypnotherapist has a problem. His stage work involves a considerable amount of travelling around the country and this will have a considerable effect upon his availability to his patients. One of the ways they have found round this is to use video-recorders as a means of recording their "therapies". This, of course, means that individual treatment is out of the question. A "standard" treatment is recorded on the tape and this is played to all patients, so there can be no variation to cater for individual needs.

Another disadvantage here is that because of their inadequacy as therapists, they often resort to aversion therapy, which was discussed earlier. Consequently, their success rate is low.

Where a stage hypnotist does not use video, he finds his availability to his patients is very much subject to his stage commitments. Consequently, a patient in, say, London will find his appointment changed because the "therapist" has a theatrical booking in Blackpool. Patients therefore take second place to the theatre. This, coupled with the lack of expertise on the part of the hypnotist does not offer much in the way of hope to a patient with a problem.

How then does one find a good therapist? Most therapists, being in full-time private practice, have to advertise. This is how you begin your search. You look in your local paper, usually under "Personal Services". There, you may find two or three to choose from. However, caution is needed here because those adverts will have been carefully worded. What follows, therefore, are a few guidelines which may be helpful when you read these adverts.

Advertising in papers is theoretically governed by the dictates of the Advertising Standards Authority. On the subject of hypnotherapy, the A.S.A. has ruled that the only treatments that can be advertised are for smoking and slimming, and apart from that, only business-card details can be included.

Unfortunately, many newspapers are not too careful about this ruling, and they will often allow therapists to advertise other conditions such as confidence, migraine, etc. The reason for this may be that the staff of the newspaper are unaware of the ruling. But regardless of this, the therapist should be aware of it. On any reputable training course for therapists the rules of advertising are carefully covered. Any advertiser who breaks these rules has either not received proper training, or has a complete disregard for codes of conduct. This then is your first clue.

Some therapists also like to create an impression by giving themselves titles and/or following their names with a string of letters. In both cases you can be misled, as you will see from the following points.

It is not uncommon for therapists to advertise themselves

as "Hypnotherapist/Psychologist". Often, the word "Psychologist" is added because it sounds good and not because they are qualified as psychologists. If they are indeed psychologists, then this will be reflected in the qualifications which follow the name. A true psychologist is a person who has at least one post-graduate qualification in Psychology. This means that they should either have Ph.D., M.A. or M.Sc. after their name. They should also be members of the British Psychological Society, which is not usually advertised as a qualification, and something you can therefore enquire about. If any of these are missing, they are not qualified to call themselves psychologists.

If qualifications are advertised, it is always good to ask about them. A good therapist will not mind explaining his qualifications to you. However, if you see qualifications like B.A. or B.Sc., then you also need to know which subject they refer to. For instance, a B.Sc. in metallurgy is of no relevance to hypnotherapy. So check on this too.

Ultimately, of course, academic qualifications are of little relevance to the subject of hypnotherapy, since there is no such thing as a degree in Hypnotherapy. The main concern therefore centres around the organisation they belong to, and this is reflected in just one set of letters which follow the name.

In the U.K., there are several organisations to which hypnotherapists belong. It will have been noticed that at the beginning of this chapter, two such organisations were mentioned by name, the reason being that in the opinion of the author, these are the only two that are worthy of note.

The I.C.H. is an organisation that sets high standards, and is not just concerned with academic knowledge. It has a good code of ethics and practice, which are designed to protect the patient. Regular seminars and workshops are held, which the entire membership is invited to attend. At these seminars, information from therapists from all over the country is pooled in order that all may be kept up-to-date with the latest techniques. The I.C.H. also provides extensive training for new therapists.

The N.C.P. is also an organisation that maintains reasonably high standards. Its members are trained in psychological analysis and the application of hypnosis. Again, membership does not just depend upon academic knowledge. New members are required to provide good character references, and agree to maintain a good code of ethics and practice. This obviously serves as a protection for its clientele. Annual conferences are held, and an internal magazine is published, through which its members are kept up-to-date with new developments in the field.

These organisations have many facilities at their disposal from which their members can benefit, but their main reason for existence is to protect the patient and to protect the good name of hypnotherapy from the threat provided by dabblers and charlatans.

Members of these two organisations have the letters "M.I.C.H.", or "M.N.C.P." after their names. With such therapists, patients are reasonably assured of good treatment.

While these two organisations have been singled out as special, it should not be taken as meaning that a good training in hypnotherapy cannot be found elsewhere. The Blythe Tutorial College of Hypnosis and Psychotherapy, for instance, runs an extremely good course in the techniques and ethics of hypnotherapy. Many doctors who use hypnosis were in fact trained there.

If you are a person who feels that you could benefit from hypnotherapy, there is enough information here to at least help you to begin to narrow the field of possibilities. You may even have selected one or two possibilities to follow up, and may now be in a position to make your enquiry. What follows is how to proceed from there.

Firstly, check out the qualifications that are advertised.

Make sure that they are relevant. Then ask about the treatment. It does not matter what you require treatment for, *you need personal attention*. Whatever you do, do not go to a therapist who will leave you in the care of a machine, like a video-recorder, because it can be dangerous and the treatment has more likelihood of failure than of success. Many conditions cannot be treated in this way. So do not be fooled. You MUST have the therapist there, to watch over you and check your progress. An underling will not do. You need to be treated as an individual in order to achieve success.

Having got this far, you may then actually go along to the practice in order to discuss your problem with the therapist. It is at this preliminary interview that you can size up your own feelings about the therapist. A good therapist will listen, ask questions, make notes, and generally discuss your problem, so that he clearly understands it. He will then decide whether or not he can treat you. If he decides to accept your case, he will then explain the procedures carefully to you, so that you know exactly what to expect. If, after this discussion, you feel happy with your choice of therapist, then go ahead with the treatment. If, however, you feel an instinctive dislike towards him, then follow that instinct and look again, because your own feelings towards him could make you resist the suggestions he gives you under hypnosis.

It is hoped that these few snippets of information will be of value to you if you find yourself in a position where you need treatment. I hope this will never be the case. Either way, having read this book, you will have a clearer idea of what hypnotherapy is and how it can be of use to you.

Some Useful Addresses

The Institute of Curative Hypnotherapists
49–51, London Road, Waterlooville
Hampshire PO7 7EX

The National Council of Psychotherapists
1, Clovelly Road, Ealing
London, W5

Blythe Tutorial College of Hypnosis
and Psychotherapy
163, Brownside Road, Worsthorne
Burnley, Lancs BB10 3JW